"A comprehensive and well-written guide that's easy to understand. It's a must-read for women of all ages looking to take charge of their heart health."

— Leslie Beck, registered dietitian, *Globe and Mail* columnist, and best-selling author of *The Complete Nutrition Guide for Women*

"A masterful summary of all we need to know about the leading killer of women, heart disease. This book should be required reading for all health conscious women and the people who love them."

— Henry Black, MD, Past President of the American Society of Hypertension, Professor of Medicine at New York University

"What a wonderful, easy to understand, comprehensive guide for living healthfully! The authors beautifully explain the importance of taking care of our most vital organ."

— Kim Coles, actor and television host

"If you have a heart and care about a woman who has a heart, you must have this book and share it with everyone you know."

— Jesse Dylan, award-winning health journalist, author and radio host of *The Good Life*

"Amazingly thorough! Written from women's hearts for women's hearts. This is a book about being aware, and it is a must for every woman's self-care library."

— Barbara Goodman, editorial director of *Canadian Health & Lifestyle* magazine

"The authors present thoughtful and practical advice that captures what every woman needs to know about her heart and how to keep it healthy."

— Alice K. Jacobs, MD, Professor of Medicine, Boston University School of Medicine

"Interesting, provocative and empowering. This book is a call to action for women to address our number one health threat."

— Fanny Kiefer, television host of *Studio 4*

"Never before has there been so great a need to educate our world on women's heart disease. *Saving Women's Hearts* will save lives and protect families from unnecessary devastation and loss."

— Danielle Lin, certified nutritionist and radio host of *The Danielle Lin Show*

"This book truly empowers women. It cuts through all the misinformation and supplies what is scientifically valid in an understandable, interesting form. I will recommend it to my patients and viewers."

— Mary Ann Malloy, MD, cardiologist and contributor to NBC Chicago

"A must-read for women of all ages. The authors provide valuable guidance on how to reduce your risk of heart disease. This book and its strategies could really save your life."

— Lynn Martin, radio host on AM800 CKLW

"*Saving Women's Hearts* is a thorough, practical, scientifically based book to empower women to conquer heart disease. The best part is that it takes so much information and makes it easy to understand."

— Jennifer H. Mieres, MD, FACC, FAHA, Associate Professor of Medicine, North Shore -LIJ School of Medicine, co-author of *Heart Smart For Black Women and Latinas*

"This book is like having a heart-to-heart with a doctor who is also your best friend. It gives practical, real-life advice about heart disease and how to prevent it."

— Aphrodite Salas, journalist

"Truly the best book on the subject. It focuses on the person, the soul, and the importance of heart health. Other books have focused on quick fixes and not applied an emotional side to getting healthy. This book takes a very female approach to a very challenging issue."

— Leslee Shaw, PhD, FACC, FAHA, FASNC, Professor of Medicine, Emory University

"Imagine a book that combines the best in conventional, natural, and complementary approaches. Imagine a book that honors pure science and the incredible advances in medical technology but also wholeheartedly accepts the brilliance of nature's offerings. You're holding that book! Don't let it go. It may save your life."

— Bryce Wylde, HD, RNC, author of *The Antioxidant Prescription*, television host of *Wylde on Health*

SAVING WOMEN'S HEARTS

How You Can Prevent and Reverse Heart Disease
With Natural and Conventional Strategies

MARTHA GULATI MD, MS, FACC, FAHA

SHERRY TORKOS BSc Phm

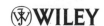

John Wiley & Sons Canada, Ltd.

Library and Archives Canada Cataloguing in Publication
Gulati, Martha, 1969–
    Saving women's hearts : how you can prevent and reverse heart disease with natural and conventional strategies / Martha Gulati, Sherry Torkos.

Includes bibliographical references and index.
ISBN 978-0-470-67845-9
978-0-470-67846-6 (e-PDF), 978-0-47067848-0 (Mobi), 978-0-47067847-3 (ePub)

    1. Heart diseases in women—Popular works. 2. Heart—Diseases—Prevention—3. Women—Diseases—Prevention—Popular works. I. Torkos, Sherry II. Title.

RC682.G84 2011   616.1'205082   C2010-906240-X

Production Credits
Cover design: Diana Sullada
Interior design and typesetting: Mike Chan
Author photos: Danny Clark Photography (M.G.)
    and Precious LaPlante Photography (S.T.)
Printer: Solisco Tri-Graphic Printing Ltd.

Editorial Credits
Managing Editor: Alison Maclean
Production Editor: Lindsay Humphreys
Editorial Assistant: Katie Wolsley

John Wiley & Sons Canada, Ltd.
6045 Freemont Blvd.
Mississauga, Ontario
L5R 4J3

Printed in Canada
1 2 3 4 5 SOL TRI 15 14 13 12 11

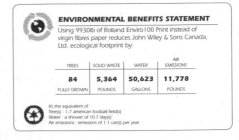

ENVIRONMENTAL BENEFITS STATEMENT
Using 9930lb of Rolland Enviro100 Print instead of virgin fibres paper reduces John Wiley & Sons Canada, Ltd. ecological footprint by:

TREES	SOLID WASTE	WATER	AIR EMISSIONS
84	5,364	50,623	11,778
FULLY GROWN	POUNDS	GALLONS	POUNDS

It's the equivalent of :
Tree(s) : 1.7 american football field(s)
Water : a shower of 10.7 day(s)
Air emissions : emissions of 1.1 car(s) per year

To the two women whose hearts I care about the most — Patricia Gulati-Conti and Natasha Conti.

To my teacher, who was the first to make me aware that women's hearts were special, Dr. Leonard Sternberg.

In memory of my mentor, who made it possible for me to do research on women's hearts, Dr. Morton Arnsdorf.

To my father, who has cheered me on in every step and is essential to my heart.

And in memory of my mother, who taught me how to use my heart.
M.G.

To my parents, who inspire me with their boundless energy and passion for life. You have led by example and taught me from an early age how to live a heart-healthy lifestyle.

To my husband Rick and baby Phoenix, I love you with all my heart.
S.T.

We dedicate this book to all the women we love and to all our patients who have entrusted us to help them save their hearts.
M.G. & S.T.

Contents

Acknowledgments

I would like to first acknowledge my brother, Justin Gulati. Hopefully he forgives me for not dedicating the book to him but he has been my biggest advocate and was the first person to tell me I should write a book on this topic. Thank you for all your great ideas (particularly the survey!), editing suggestions, and being my greatest fan. I also must thank my sister Patricia Gulati. Thank you for walking around Southern Florida making random women fill out my survey! I am sorry you couldn't give them the answers on the spot, but it was your friends and contacts that helped us learn what women needed to know and helped us shape the book. So thank you to all of the women who took the survey, too. My father has always been my biggest fan and will be forcing both women *and men* to read this book, because he is my dad. Thanks for your unconditional love. I would also like to acknowledge the constant support and feedback from my friends and family as we wrote the book. Thank you to Gareth Gwyn for your love, patience, and for always being on my side (even when I may be wrong!). I must also thank Christine Pauley-Kultgen. Without you as my friend, I would have never met your mom who is "being forced to exercise more every time a new set of guidelines comes out." In addition, without you, my vocabulary would be incomplete.

I would particularly like to thank the Peggy Shure-Snyder family, the Nancy and Larry Glick family, and the Sally and Bill Soter family for supporting my work and my research on women.

I am also grateful for the support and shaping of my career from the following people: Drs. Leonard Sternberg, Arthur Rubenstein, Morton Arnsdorf, Jeffery Lieden, Henry Black, Noel Bairey-Merz, Leslee Shaw, Jennifer Mieres, Robert Bonow, Neil Stone, Tom Ryan, William Abraham, and Nanette Wenger.

To all my patients who I have had the honor of taking care of, please know this book was shaped by the questions you asked and the things I learned from you. You continue to be my inspiration and my daily joy.

Thanks to the Wiley team for helping us with the book and believing in our idea, particularly Leah Fairbank for being the best advocate for us and getting our book off the ground. Thank you also to our lawyer and family friend, Mr. John Burns, for the legal guidance.

Lastly, I must thank my co-author, Sherry Torkos, who has been a friend since the first day in university freshman year where we found we were in the same calculus and physics classes. One of us loved the classes, one did not, so we were a bit like protons and electrons, don't you think? Our strengths continue to complement each other, even our career paths. Your optimism, patience, and passion are always an inspiration to me. Your ability to work on this book during a crazy year ending with Baby Phoenix was a stress test of its own. You passed with flying colors, dear friend. You are part of my heart for life.

Martha Gulati

There are many people I would like to thank for their help and support with this book.

To my husband Rick and my family: thank you for your encouragement, patience, and understanding of my commitment to this project and all the long hours required to see it through.

To my coauthor, Martha: I am so grateful for the opportunity to work with you on this book. I admire your vast knowledge and expertise and your dedication to research and the advancement of our understanding of heart disease and women. I also value your friendship. We have had many fun times together. From the days when we were studying science together at McMaster University and through the many twists and turns our lives have taken, you have always been a true friend.

To the team at Wiley: Leah Fairbank, Alison Maclean, Lindsay Humphreys, and the sales and marketing teams, thanks for all your help and support with this book.

Finally, I would like to thank you, the reader, for your interest and for taking the time to read this book. I sincerely hope that this information empowers you to take care of your heart.

Sherry Torkos

Heart Disease in Women

Wherever you go, go with all your heart.
— Confucius

Why should you care about your heart? Why does your heart matter at *any* age? Well, heart disease is the number-one killer of women. Most women think cancer (particularly breast cancer) should be their number-one health concern, but the facts are the facts. One out of three women will develop heart disease in her lifetime.[1] And we are more likely to die of heart disease as adults than we are to die from the next six leading causes of death. But heart disease is the single most preventable cause of death, which means we can change the odds of getting this disease that claims too many women's lives every year.

Given the statistics, all of us must think about our hearts, take care of our hearts, watch our hearts, and know our hearts. It is never too late or too early to start and to make changes to reduce your risk of heart disease. All women need to be proactive about knowing their risks for heart disease and working to reduce those risks.

You may ask yourself why this book should matter to you, especially if you don't have heart disease or don't identify yourself as being at risk for heart disease. The truth is, most women do not recognize themselves as being at risk for heart disease. Women are less likely than men to recognize symptoms of a heart attack, which are often different for women than they are for men, and less likely to call an ambulance or 9-1-1 when they are having symptoms of an attack.[2] As a result, we women are more likely to delay getting care when we are having a heart attack. And not only do heart attacks in women frequently go unnoticed by the women themselves but they are often unrecognized by their doctors. Even after a heart attack is diagnosed, women are less likely to leave the hospital with the standard medications (as per national guidelines for anyone with a heart attack, regardless of gender) that have proven to save lives. This ultimately leads to higher death rates for women, and particularly younger women, which is very concerning.[3] We need to change this. Although the risk for a woman to get heart disease in her lifetime is one in three, it will soon be one in two if the trends keep going in the direction we are seeing. That means that the odds of you getting heart disease are the same as getting heads in a coin toss — not great odds for any woman.

To help stack those odds in your favor, we decided to write this book, in which we give you information that you can incorporate into your daily life to reduce your risk of heart disease and stroke. We come at this topic from different angles. One of us is a pharmacist, with training in both conventional and complementary medicine. One of us is a cardiologist specializing in cardiac disease prevention in women and who does research on heart disease prevention in women. But, first and foremost, *we are both women*. We are passionate about this issue and have our own personal reasons for wanting to reduce heart disease in women: we both have family histories that predispose us to developing heart disease. We've chosen to devote ourselves to learning as much as possible about our hearts and how to protect them, so that we can take care of our hearts and help other women, like you, do the same.

While we were doing our respective schooling and training, we were both shocked to discover how little was known about women and heart disease. And we are not talking about so long ago — this was the mid-1990s. Naively, we thought that most of medicine was well studied, and that, in particular, the number-one killer of women should be! But to our amazement, we found that women were routinely excluded from most of the major cardiology trials. So the medicine we were practicing took for granted that women are the same as men — that they would present in the same way and respond to medications in the same way, that their disease patterns for heart disease would be identical to men, and that the tests used to diagnose heart disease would work equally as well in women as men, even if they were not tested or validated in women. But these were assumptions, not facts. And the fact is this: until the 1990s, few women were even included in large cardiology trials, so we really did not know very much about women and heart disease.

It is amazing that the medical field did not recognize this for such a long time. Heart disease was killing women across the globe. Women had worse outcomes after a heart attack, worse outcomes after undergoing heart surgery, and since 1984 more women were dying from heart disease than men. Dr. Nanette Wenger, a cardiologist from Emory University and the former chief of Grady Hospital in Atlanta who really led the movement for cardiac research in women, said it best: "The [medical] community has viewed women's health almost with a 'bikini' approach, looking essentially at the breast and reproductive system, and almost ignoring the rest of the woman as part of women's health."[4]

When we spoke of women's health, we were talking about fertility and reproductive health, breast cancer, and ovarian disease. But not the heart. The good news for all women is that we have come such a long way since then. We have made huge strides in the last 15 or more years. The U.S. government mandated that women be included in all new clinical trials, and the largest study of women and hormone replacement therapy (the U.S.-based Women's Health Initiative) was started as a result of that mandate. We now have evidence-based guidelines for heart disease prevention in women. We are studying the effects of medications on women, as well as the side effects, and determining the appropriate dosing for women. Because of the National Institutes of Health mandate, we have more trials that include both women and men, and we are able to compare gender differences in heart disease. We are tracking how well women do after a heart attack and after coronary bypass surgery. And since 2001, we have seen a decline in mortality in women from heart disease.[5] So we are definitely making progress; but we are nowhere close to having all the answers or completing all the trials that will tell us for certain what methods of prevention and treatment work best for women and heart disease.

Despite the inclusion of women in heart studies and the like, heart disease is still considered to be a "man's disease." Women need to be aware that it is, however, an equal opportunity aggressor. It just announces itself about 10 years earlier in men, but once it affects women, it is a whole lot tougher: More women than men die of heart disease each year. Women are more likely to die from a heart attack than a man. More women than men die within one year of having a heart attack. Twice as many women than men end up disabled as a result of heart disease.

We are writing this book to guide you through today's best evidence of what will help you save your heart. We want women to recognize that they are at risk for heart disease and that it is the number-one killer of women. We want to present you with the tools to do everything you can to prevent getting heart disease. And for those women with heart disease, we want to help protect you from any future problems and equip you with the tools to maintain the healthiest heart possible. We want all women to be aware of the symptoms of heart disease and to know what to do when you think you may be having a heart attack. In this book we will tell you about the most recent studies on women and heart disease prevention, so that you can make informed decisions about how to keep you and your heart healthy. We want you to know what kind of heart testing and screening you need, and what to expect when you get tests done. We will present you with evidence-based treatment options, regardless of whether we are discussing conventional Western medications or complementary medicines. We want all women to feel empowered to understand their hearts so they can have frank, informed discussions with their healthcare providers about what needs to be done for their own individual hearts.

Survey of What Women Know About Their Hearts

Before we decided to write this book, we performed a survey to find out what women know about their health and their hearts. This survey is copied below. Why don't you go ahead and take it now? We'll discuss the results in the final chapter.

Pompano Beach Heart Survey

1. What is your number-one health concern?
   A. Breast cancer
   B. Cervical cancer
   C. Lung disease
   D. Heart disease
   E. Mental illness
   F. Other

2. What is the number-one killer of women?
   A. Breast cancer
   B. Cervical cancer
   C. Lung cancer
   D. Heart disease
   E. Suicide

3. Have you ever been screened for heart disease?
   A. Yes
   B. No

4. Do you think you are at risk for heart disease?
   A. Yes
   B. No

5. What is the lifetime risk of heart disease?
   A. One in three women will develop heart disease in their lifetime.
   B. One in 100 women will develop heart disease in their lifetime.
   C. One in 1000 women will develop heart disease in their lifetime.
   D. One in 10,000 women will develop heart disease in their lifetime.

6. Which supplement is recommended for heart disease prevention?
   A. Folic acid
   B. Vitamin E
   C. Vitamin C
   D. Fish oil (omega-3)
   E. Beta-carotene

7. What is normal blood pressure?
   A. Less than 100/70
   B. Less than 120/80
   C. Less than 135/85
   D. Less than 140/90

8. What is normal body mass index (BMI)?
   A. $<25 \, kg/m^2$
   B. $<30 \, kg/m^2$
   C. $<35 \, kg/m^2$
   D. I am unaware of what the body mass index is.

9. Which supplement should all women take daily to prevent heart disease?
   A. Aspirin (81 mg)
   B. Aspirin (325 mg)
   C. Folate
   D. None of the above
   E. All of the above

10. Which of the following are risk factors for heart disease in women?
    A. Tobacco use
    B. Physical inactivity
    C. Family history of heart disease
    D. All of the above
    E. None of the above

11. At what age should women be screened for heart disease?
    A. Age 60 and above
    B. Age 50 and above
    C. Age 40 and above
    D. Age 30 and above
    E. Age 20 and above

12. After a woman under the age of 60 has a heart attack, she is more likely to survive compared to a man of the same age who has a heart attack.
    A. Yes
    B. No

13. Does hormone replacement therapy protect women against heart disease?
    A. Yes
    B. No

14. How informed about heart disease do you feel you are?
    A. Poorly informed
    B. Moderately informed
    C. Highly informed

Chapter 1

Affairs of a Woman's Heart

And now here is my secret, a very simple secret;
it is only with the heart that one can see rightly,
what is essential is invisible to the eye.
— Antoine de Saint Exupery

Think of your heart as a muscle. No, wait, let's use an analogy, one that all women can relate to. Think of your heart as your favorite pair of shoes. Whether you love them for their comfort or for their style, they are your favorite shoes and you wonder if you could ever replace them if they wore out. You know which shoes we are talking about — the ones you wish you'd had the foresight to buy multiple pairs of. So you treat those shoes with great care and love, because you want them to last forever. Wearing the right pair of shoes can make you feel amazing, like you can conquer all your problems and, well, just deal a little better with life in general.

The same can be said for a healthy heart. But unlike a pair of shoes, the heart is hidden from view, so you don't think about it all the time. You may not even think about it at all when it is working well. And when it's not working well, you may become more familiar with it, but by then it may be too late.

Remember that we each get one heart and one heart only, so it's imperative that we treat it well. So let's start thinking about our hearts every time we put on a pair of shoes, which, for most of us, is at least once a day.

In this chapter, we introduce you to the heart and all its parts. We describe how the heart functions normally and what can go wrong in the heart.

What Is Your Heart?

The heart is a muscle. Quite an amazing muscle, in fact. Its two sides are not exactly the same, but similar, and they work in unison. One side cannot work without the other. The top chambers on the left and right sides are called the *atria*. The bottom chambers (again one on the right side, one on the left) are called the *ventricles*. You can see the different parts of the heart in the diagram below.

Anatomy of Your Heart

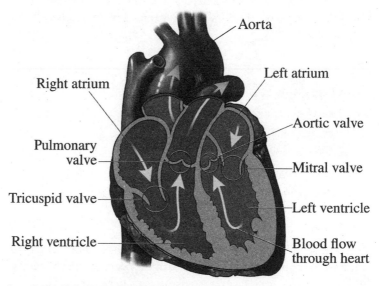

The atria and ventricles work in coordination. When the ventricles relax and fill with blood, the atria contract; and when the atria relax and fill, the ventricles contract and pump the blood forward — to the *aorta* on the left side and to the *pulmonary arteries* on the right side. The aorta is the largest artery in the body, originating at the exit of the heart, and from the aorta, all the other arteries branch off to provide blood to all the organs and tissues in the body. The pulmonary arteries carry the venous blood from the right side of the heart to the lungs to get oxygen and return this blood to the left side of the heart through the pulmonary veins.

The ventricles are the real powerhouses of the heart, particularly the left ventricle. If you look at the ventricles, you will see the thick muscle that makes up this chamber. In a normal heart, the left ventricle is more muscular than the right. Nonetheless, both ventricles handle the same volume of blood, so the right side of the heart is just as important as the left side.

The left and right sides of the heart are separate, meaning they do not exchange any blood directly across the atria or ventricles. If they do transfer blood between any of these chambers, there is likely a hole in the heart and this is abnormal. Normally, the heart keeps the venous blood (blood that has been depleted of its oxygen) from the right side of the heart separate from the oxygenated blood in the left side of the heart.

Did you know . . .

The heart beats approximately

♥ 70 beats a minute

♥ 10,000 beats a day

♥ 38 million beats a year

♥ 2.5 billion times over 70 years

The atria fill with blood from the venous systems that empty on both sides of the heart, but the right side of the heart gets the blood that has had most of its oxygen extracted and is returning from the body. The right side of the heart pumps the blood through the pulmonary artery to get oxygen from the lungs, and it returns the blood to the left side of the heart through the *pulmonary veins*, where the blood is now rich with oxygen. The left side of the heart pumps the blood through the aorta. This blood, now rich in oxygen, goes to all of the arteries in the body, including those that supply the heart muscle.

You can understand how if the heart can't work, meaning if it can't pump blood to the body, the rest of the body can't work. We need our hearts to function, otherwise all the other organs of the body will fail to get blood and, therefore, the oxygen they need to do their jobs. Ultimately this will cause all the organs to shut down and stop working. This is why the heart is the most important organ in the body. Without a working heart, we cannot live.

The Coronary Arteries

The coronary arteries provide the blood supply to the heart. These arteries get their blood supply every time the heart beats. Each time the left ventricle pumps blood forward through the aorta, the coronary arteries fill and provide the muscle of the heart with oxygen-rich blood so that the heart can work.

What Can Go Wrong with the Heart Arteries?

The heart muscle requires a constant supply of oxygen to function and this oxygen comes through the heart arteries. If the heart arteries are blocked, and thus the blood flow to the heart muscle is blocked or severely reduced, oxygen will not get to the heart muscle and the muscle can be damaged. This is what occurs when someone has a heart attack — also known as a *myocardial infarction* or, if you watch television medical dramas, an "MI." (We discuss heart attacks in more detail in Chapter 6.) A myocardial infarction is the most common cause of heart disease in women, so we really want you to understand exactly how this occurs and how you can prevent it and treat it.

The coronary arteries can become blocked over time due to a gradual buildup of plaque, made up primarily of cholesterol. This process is known as *atherosclerosis.* If the cholesterol plaque ruptures or breaks in response to stress, a blood clot can form and block the artery completely, preventing blood from flowing forward to the area beyond the blockage. Since the heart muscle past the blockage is dependent on that artery for its oxygen supply, a blockage in blood flow will damage it. This condition of the heart muscle not receiving enough oxygen to function properly is known as *ischemia.* If the blood flow is not quickly restored, that affected area of the heart muscle may die (*infarct*).

Less common problems with the coronary arteries may be the result of birth defects in the heart artery anatomy, for example, congenital abnormalities in the positions of the coronary arteries. Such an abnormality may require surgical correction if the artery position results in compression of the artery, which would ultimately lead to ischemia, even when there is no plaque buildup. *Vasospasm*, where the heart artery contracts and reduces the blood flow to the heart muscle, is another problem.

The Heart Valves

The heart's four valves keep the blood flowing in the appropriate direction. These valves are made up of *leaflets (triangular-like flaps)*. The heart valves open and close within the heart cycle, allowing the blood to flow in one direction only: forward. When the valves are working normally they open and close fully and at appropriate times when the heart contracts. The heart valves between the atria and ventricles are known as the *tricuspid valve* and *mitral valve*, on the right and left side of the heart, respectively; the valve between the right ventricle and the pulmonary artery is the *pulmonic valve*; and the valve between the left ventricle and the aorta is called the *aortic valve*. Refer to the diagram of the heart on page 9 to see the position of the heart valves.

What Can Go Wrong with Heart Valves?

Two things can potentially go wrong with heart valves. First, they can leak and allow blood to flow backwards. This is known as *regurgitation* and can occur with any of the four valves. Second, the valves can become tight and narrow, making it difficult for blood to flow forward. This is known as *stenosis,* and it, too, can affect any of the four valves. In addition, more than one valve can be affected by the same disease process, and a person can have a leaky valve and tight valve at the same time.

Regurgitation and stenosis may be caused by congenital valve problems (that is, you are born with them), infections of the heart valves, rheumatic fever affecting the heart valves, damage to a heart valve or its structure after a heart attack or after developing heart failure, or valve disease from aging where there is calcification on the valves.

Symptoms are important signals, but changes to the heart can occur even without symptoms. If the valve is not repaired or replaced, more damage to the heart may occur, depending on how much the disease process affects the heart valves' ability to open or close (or both) properly. Heart function can start declining as a result of the valve problem and, if left untreated, may be irreversible.

The Heart Ventricles

The ventricles of the heart are in charge of pumping the nutrient-rich blood to the body and its organs, providing adequate nourishment and oxygen to all the organs so that they can function normally.

What Can Go Wrong with the Heart Ventricles?

When the ventricles of the heart are not working normally, the heart cannot pump blood as effectively as it should. When our heart cannot meet the body's demands, we are said to have *heart failure*. Even though the term may imply that the heart can't work at all, it can just not as well as a healthy heart. There is a remarkable spectrum of severity of this disease. Some people with heart failure have no symptoms at all, while others are so limited by their heart failure that the simple act of moving about their home can be difficult. Heart failure can occur even when the heart function appears normal but the heart cannot relax normally; this is known as *diastolic heart failure* and is common in women.

Heart failure can result from several causes, including a heart attack or *coronary artery disease* (where one or more of the coronary arteries is narrowed), hypertension, valve disorders, chemotherapy drugs, alcohol, or infections or disease processes that affect the heart muscle.

> Each year, 267,000 U.S. women die from heart attacks, which kill six times as many women as breast cancer. Another 31,837 women die each year of congestive heart failure, representing 62.6% of all heart failure deaths.

The Electrical System of the Heart

What is really fascinating about the heart is that it has its own electrical system that responds to your body's demands and requirements, telling the heart when to beat faster or slower, depending on how active you are. If you suddenly break into a run, your heart knows: your heart rate picks up. When you stop running, it knows it can safely and gradually slow down. When you sleep, the body's demands for blood and oxygen lessen, so the heart slows down its rate even further from your resting heart rate of your waking hours.

It is the *sinoatrial node* (SA node or sinus node) located in the right atrium that usually controls the heart rate. When working properly, the SA node generates an electrical signal that then moves from the right atrium to the left atrium and on to the *atrioventricular node* (AV node), where through a specialized conduction system (*His-Purkinje system*) the electrical impulse is transferred to the ventricles. It is this electrical impulse that causes the heart to pump. If it is disrupted anywhere along this pathway, the heart rhythm may be affected, as well as the normal functioning of the heart.

If for some reason the sinoatrial node fails, many other places in the heart can take over. Basically, every cell that makes up the heart muscle is capable of sending a charge or signal to help keep the heart beating. Which part of the heart takes control determines the heart rate.

What Can Go Wrong with the Heart's Electrical System?

Arrhythmias, irregular or abnormal heartbeats, are quite common and can range from inconsequential to life-threatening. Arrhythmias are more common as we age. We discuss in more detail the different rhythm disorders later, but briefly, your heart can beat too quickly (*tachycardia*), too slowly (*bradycardia*), or too early (either *premature atrial contractions* or PACs, or *premature ventricular contractions* or PVCs), which can feel like a skipped beat. Arrhythmias can be regular or irregular. Some arrhythmias may occur unnoticed — you only learn about them through a doctor's exam or when an electrocardiogram is performed. Some arrhythmias require no treatment at all, some require medications, some require a pacemaker to regulate the heart rate, and some require immediate defibrillation to shock the heart to bring about a more stable rhythm. Some arrhythmias require an implanted defibrillator that will shock the heart when it detects that a dangerous arrhythmia is occurring.

Cardiac arrest, when the heart stops working, is the most dangerous of all arrhythmias. Usually this occurs because of *ventricular fibrillation,* when the ventricles have electrical activity but it is too fast for the ventricles to effectively pump blood, and so blood circulation ceases. This may be a consequence of a heart attack, but there are other causes as well.

The Pericardium

The *pericardium* is a thin-membrane sac surrounding the heart. As well as containing the heart, it contains the roots of the *great vessels* (the aorta, pulmonary artery, pulmonary vein, and the vena cava). The pericardium has two layers — like a sac within a sac — separated by a space known as the *pericardial space,* which is filled with a thin amount of lubricant, the *pericardial fluid.*

What Can Go Wrong with the Pericardium?

Pericarditis, or inflammation of the pericardium, can occur after a certain type of infection. It can also occur after a heart attack, after heart surgery, or after radiation treatment to the chest area. It also can result from cancer in organs near the heart (the lungs, the breast, the blood system). Pericarditis may occur after certain trauma or injuries to the chest area. It is seen, too, with autoimmune disorders (like lupus or rheumatoid arthritis) or in persons with kidney failure. Rarely, this can occur with exposure to toxic fumes. When pericarditis is present, a person will often experience chest pain that can be sharp and can get worse when changing position or when taking deep breaths. This inflammation can result in an increase in the amount of pericardial fluid, known as a *pericardial effusion.*

Pericardial effusion can also result without pericarditis in those with heart failure, kidney failure, certain cancers (particularly breast and lung cancer), or because of hypothyroidism. It may be seen in people after heart surgery or after chest injuries or trauma, where blood accumulates in the pericardial space. If the amount of fluid collected in the pericardium becomes so large that it affects the ability of the heart to function, the result is *pericardial tamponade,* which is life-threatening. If tamponade is diagnosed, the fluid in this space needs to be removed as quickly as possible.

The Circulatory System

The blood from the heart is delivered to the body through the arterial system that starts at the *aorta*, the artery that sits just above the heart to which the ventricle pumps blood. The aorta is the largest artery in the body. From this large vessel that goes up toward the top of the body and then arches downward, numerous arteries branch off to even smaller arterioles, creating a *capillary bed* that brings the oxygen and nutrients to all the organs, muscles, and tissues in the body. When the heart is included in this *circulatory system*, it is known as the *cardiovascular system*. The cardiovascular system includes the heart, the coronary arteries, and the entire arterial system of the body.

What Can Go Wrong with the Circulation?

A *stroke* occurs when there is disease in the arteries to the brain, causing a reduction in the blood supply to the brain. Stroke is the third leading cause of death and can occur at any age, although most (three-quarters of all strokes) occur in people over the age of 65. There are two types of stroke. The most common type of stroke is an *ischemic stroke,* which accounts for 87% of all strokes. An ischemic stroke occurs when a blood clot (*thrombus*) blocks the blood flow in an artery to an area of the brain. This is often the result of plaque buildup in the arteries, or atherosclerosis, the same disease that can occur in the heart arteries, as described earlier. This is why heart disease and ischemic stroke are often discussed together: Although the organs affected are different, the diseases are the result of the same process and the same risk factors. Another cause of ischemic stroke is a blood clot that has formed elsewhere (usually in the heart) and lodges in an artery that supplies the brain. It can develop in the heart as a result of atrial fibrillation because the heart cannot pump efficiently and blood pools in the atria, creating a clot. A clot may also form in women who use hormonal contraceptives and who smoke, which can result in a stroke.

The other type of stroke is a *hemorrhagic stroke.* Here, too, the blood to the brain tissue is reduced, but this is a result of an artery to the brain bursting or rupturing, causing a bleed around the brain tissue. This is less common and is not a result of atherosclerosis, but rather it is caused by an abnormality of the blood vessel in the brain. These blood vessels can be aggravated by high blood pressure, but risk factors responsible for coronary artery disease and ischemic stroke do not cause a hemorrhagic stroke.

The facts about women and stroke

- ♥ Stroke is the third leading cause of death in women, following heart disease and cancer.
- ♥ Every year, stroke kills twice as many women as breast cancer.
- ♥ The risk of a stroke in women doubles each decade after the age of 55.
- ♥ Every year in the United States, about 55,000 more women than men have a stroke, and women are more likely to die from a stroke than men.
- ♥ A smoker has double the risk of having an ischemic stroke than a nonsmoker.
- ♥ Physical activity is associated with a lower risk of stroke.

Peripheral vascular disease, also known as *peripheral arterial disease* (PAD), is the result of progressive plaque formation in the arteries (narrowing of the arteries) in the circulation system outside of the brain and the heart. It is a result of atherosclerosis, the same disease process responsible for disease of the heart and brain arteries. Risk factors that cause heart disease and stroke can also cause PAD, but there is greater risk of PAD in women who smoke or who are diabetic. If the PAD is severe, there can be a complete blockage of blood flow to the arteries, and if blood flow is not restored, the limb affected (most often the leg) will need to be amputated.

An *aortic aneurysm* is when an area of the aorta is dilated or bulging out. It often occurs as a result of atherosclerosis in the aorta (which is no different from the atherosclerosis seen elsewhere in any artery), but can also be seen in persons with Marfan Syndrome and some other disorders where the artery walls are abnormal. An aneurysm is a weak wall in that area of the aorta and is at high risk of rupturing, causing the blood to spill out of the aorta. It is also at high risk of dissecting or tearing, causing an *aortic dissection.* This is where the inner lining of the artery splits and blood flows into the lining of the artery. Both can occur anywhere along the aorta, but the condition is most dangerous when it appears in the part of the aorta coming off the heart (the *ascending aorta*). It is particularly dangerous since it may be present without any symptoms. Interestingly, aortic dissections appear to occur more frequently in men than women.

Aortic aneurysms and aortic dissections

♥ The larger the aortic aneurysm, the more likely it is to burst.

♥ Some aortic aneurysms (based on size) do not require emergent treatment but are followed with imaging over time to check if they are enlarging.

♥ The symptom of an acute aortic dissection is sudden chest pain.

♥ If they are detected, aortic aneurysms and aortic dissections can be successfully treated.

The Heart of the Matter

The heart and the cardiovascular system have complex and amazing structures. Every heartbeat keeps us alive. We rely on our hearts to function normally, so we need to be aware of them, take care them, and make sure to check them on a regular basis. Some things that can go wrong in the heart are apparent only when they do go wrong. But other problems are deceptively quiet — until it is too late. So every woman needs to know her heart and how to protect it. Remember our advice: think about your heart every time you put on your shoes. And treat your heart like your favorite pair of shoes — love it, care for it, and do everything you can to protect it. Next, we guide you on just how to protect your heart and keep it healthy, so keep reading.

Chapter 2

The Risks to a Woman's Heart

The consequences of our actions are so complicated, so diverse,
that predicting the future is a very difficult business indeed.
— J.K. Rowling, *Harry Potter and the Prisoner of Azkaban*

The question that all women need to ask is, "Am I at risk for heart disease?" That is truly an important question. And the answer is that we are all at risk for developing heart disease. As we mentioned in our Introduction, according to current statistics, a woman's risk of developing heart disease is approximately one in three, but this risk is approaching one in two. What this means for women is that the odds of developing heart disease are almost 50:50.

Nonetheless, certain risk factors put us at greater risk of getting heart disease. Therefore, it is important to know what those risk factors are and what can be done to change them to reduce the odds of having a heart attack or developing atherosclerosis. Some risk factors are *non-modifiable*, meaning you can't change them. But in truth, most risk factors for heart disease *are modifiable*, meaning you *can* change them. So, we'll show you how to change them for the better to reduce your risk of heart disease. You'll also learn which risk factors are proven to cause heart disease and for which you should be screened. Even if you already have heart disease, knowing the risk factors that contributed to your getting heart disease and knowing which you can change will help you reduce your risk of having future heart problems.

In this chapter, we also examine some of the emerging risk factors that are getting increased attention and may be related to heart disease development. Some of the emerging risk factors appear to be associated with heart disease, but if there is no proven therapy for them, while they are interesting from a scientific standpoint, their relevance remains to be proven. We want you to concentrate on the risk factors that you *can* change — those factors for which proven and effective therapies exist — so you can reduce your overall risk of heart disease. Below is a list of risk factors for developing heart disease.

Risk Factors for Heart Disease Development

Non-modifiable risk factors	Modifiable risk factors	Emerging risk factors
Age	Smoking	High-sensitivity C-reactive protein (hs-CRP)
Genetics (family history)	High blood pressure	Apolipoprotein B
Race/Ethnicity	High cholesterol	Homocysteine
	Diabetes	Fibrinogen
	Physical inactivity/Poor fitness	Lipoprotein (a)
	Metabolic syndrome	Lipoprotein subfractions
	Obesity	
	Stress, depression, and anxiety	
	Sleep apnea	
	Sleep	

Non-Modifiable Risk Factors: What You Can't Change

As we mentioned earlier, some of the risk factors for heart disease aren't things that you are able to change. In this section, we look at these factors.

Age: When It Comes to Your Heart, It Is More than Just a Number

To me, old age is always 15 years older than I am.

— Bernard M. Baruch

You can lie about your age, but you can't fool Mother Nature. Your biological age is what it is. And the older we become, the greater the risk we are at for developing heart disease. Since heart disease is the number-one killer of women, it can be present at any age, but it is more likely to be a health issue for women after the age of 55.

Our risk of developing heart disease appears to be delayed by about 10 years when compared with men. We seem to be protected in some way by our estrogen levels; however, it is unclear if the decrease in estrogen that occurs with menopause is solely responsible for all the cardiovascular changes that occur at that time. Studies that used hormone replacement therapy in postmenopausal women failed to show an improvement in cardiovascular outcomes, so the truth behind what exactly is going on is not completely clear. It is not estrogen alone that is causing the changes we see at menopause. What we do know is that as women go through menopause, many of the modifiable risk factors for heart disease start to change for the worse. And so, ultimately, the risk and occurrence of heart disease development increases during menopause.

> A major U.S. study, the Women's Health Initiative (WHI), suggests that the long-term use of HRT (estrogen plus progestin) significantly increases women's risks of heart attacks, stroke, and breast cancer.

Regardless of whether we are menstruating or not, plaque builds up over time in our arteries as we age. Just how much plaque is determined by both our lifestyles and genetics. When the plaque builds up to a point where the blood flow to the heart is reduced, we may experience symptoms of coronary artery disease because of the reduced blood flow to the heart. We can't change the fact that we age. And we can't change our genetics. But we can change our lifestyle to reduce our risk.

Genetics: Fitting into Your Genes

Genetics explains why you look like your father, and if you don't,
why you should.

— Anonymous

Like age, we can't change our family history and we can't choose our parents. At this point anyway, our genes are not modifiable. If you have a strong family history of heart disease, you are at a higher risk of heart disease.

It is a bit hard to tease out the factors about family history that may be related to developing heart disease. For example, was it the genetic makeup of DNA that caused heart disease in your family members, or was it a consequence of lifestyle or untreated risk factors that are common to your family? Doctors sometimes check a person's genetic makeup to see if the genes known to be related to heart disease are present and put that person at higher risk. But we do not yet know all the genes that might increase risk.

When doctors ask about family history for heart disease, what they want to know is if any first-degree relatives — those with whom you share the most common genetic material: your mother, father, brothers, sisters, and children — have or have had heart disease or a stroke. Doctors do, of course, care to know about more extended family members with heart disease, but if those with whom you share the most similar DNA have had heart disease, your category of risk for heart disease is considered increased.

The age at which family members have had heart disease or a stroke is also important. If several "younger" members of your family have heart disease, your risk is higher and your physician will likely be more aggressive in treating your risk factors for heart disease. "Younger" (or premature) refers to any first-degree female relative who has had a heart attack or been diagnosed with heart disease before the age of 65, and any first-degree male relative before the age of 55.

A strong family history of heart disease does not mean that you will definitely develop heart disease. What it does mean is that you may be at higher risk for it. With appropriate screening, risk factor management, and lifestyle changes, your risk can be reduced and heart disease can be prevented.

Race and Ethnicity: Who We Are and Where We Came From

You cannot put the same shoe on every foot.

— Publilius Syrus

Another non-modifiable risk factor for heart disease is race and ethnicity. Certain races and ethnic groups are at higher risk for heart disease than others, and particular races may not respond well to certain medications used to treat specific heart diseases. Of course, as our society becomes more mixed, it may be hard to pinpoint one's race and ethnicity. So if you wonder why your doctor asks about (or presumes) either, know that there is a reason for it. Below is a brief discussion of race and ethnicity as it relates to heart disease.

The age-adjusted rate of heart disease for African American women is 72% higher than for Caucasian women, and African American women ages 55 to 64 are twice as likely as Caucasian women to have a heart attack and 35% more likely to suffer from coronary artery disease.

In the United States, it is people of African descent who are at the highest risk for heart disease and who have the highest rates of heart disease, including coronary artery disease, stroke, high blood pressure, and heart failure. It is surprising and hard to accept, but women of African descent who have heart disease are twice as likely to have a heart attack and twice as likely to die from heart disease compared with their Caucasian counterparts. They appear to be less likely to get medications or treatments that could save their lives and, as a result, have the poorest prognosis once diagnosed with heart disease. African American women are more likely to have hypertension, high cholesterol, and diabetes than are their Caucasian counterparts; they are also less likely to have control of these risk factors, which is likely contributing to these disturbing outcomes. It is estimated that in the United States, 40% of African American women have some form of heart disease, in contrast with an estimated 24% of Caucasian women.

Mexican American women are also at high risk for heart disease; this is related to a very high risk of diabetes among this population. South Asians, too, are at a very high risk for heart disease; in contrast, people of Japanese descent are not. Native Americans and Native Canadians previously had low rates of heart disease, but now heart disease is a very important issue for these populations, as it is the leading cause of death among them.

Ultimately, race and ethnicity can contribute to heart disease, but this is a complex factor made up of a combination of similar genetic makeup, lifestyle, and dietary habits common among certain populations, as well as socioeconomic influences such as access to health care and quality of treatment, which influences the patterns in heart disease that we are seeing.

When it comes to heart disease risk factors, what we can't change, we must accept. What we can change, we must.

Look at the woman beside you. Statistically speaking, either you or she will develop heart disease. So when we ask, "Who is at risk?" the answer truly is "Everyone." Which means that everyone needs to know what places them at risk and how they can reduce the odds of them getting heart disease.

Modifiable Risk Factors: What You Can Change
Smoking

For women who smoke, the best way to lower your risk for a heart attack is to stop smoking. We know, easier said than done. But let's look at what we know. Smoking is the leading cause of death from cardiovascular disease — heart disease and stroke — and smoking is the leading cause of preventable deaths. Smoking cigarettes puts a person at the highest risk for heart disease, but it is believed that cigars and pipes are also associated with an increased risk of cardiovascular disease, albeit a somewhat lower risk than cigarettes. Secondhand smoke exposure is also a risk for heart disease. It is estimated that somewhere between 22,700 and 69,600 premature deaths in the United States occur from heart and blood vessel disease yearly caused by exposure to other people's smoking. In Canada, there are approximately 2,000 deaths a year from heart disease in nonsmokers due to secondhand smoke. Nonsmokers who are exposed to secondhand smoke at home or at work have a 20 to 30% increased risk for heart disease.

Secondhand smoke and your heart

♥ Secondhand smoke exposure *can* cause a heart attack.

♥ Secondhand smoke increases one's risk of coronary artery disease by 25%.

♥ Even brief exposure to secondhand smoke could trigger a heart attack.

♥ Nonsmokers have more than a 70% increased risk of stroke if they live with a smoker.

♥ Smoke-free air laws have resulted in fewer heart attacks.

When you smoke or are exposed to smoke, the toxins from the cigarettes that enter the bloodstream contribute to plaque formation on the coronary artery walls (and on the other arteries in the body), accelerating the process of atherosclerosis. Smoking can also raise blood pressure, lower the body's level of good cholesterol (HDL cholesterol, which helps to keep artery walls free of plaque), and damage the arteries. Damage to the arteries from smoking can increase the risk of peripheral artery disease and aortic aneurysms. When other risk factors are present, smoking acts with these to increase the risk of heart disease. And there's more: women smokers who use hormone-based contraceptives have a much higher risk of coronary heart disease and stroke compared with their nonsmoking counterparts. Women who smoke are advised not to take hormone-based contraceptives because of this increased risk, but many women often do, despite warnings from their doctors, pharmacists, and the drug manufacturers.

Worldwide, 8.6 million women die from heart disease each year, accounting for a third of all deaths in women. Three million women die from stroke each year. Stroke accounts for more deaths among women than men (11% vs. 8.4%) because women face the additional risk of using oral contraceptives in combination with smoking.

Although smoking rates are lower today than they were in the past, smoking continues to be the number-one preventable cause of death. In 2005, 20% of Canadian women reported being "regular smokers" (defined as either daily or occasional smokers). In the United States, 21.1 million women are regular smokers, which is about 18% of the female population. By race or ethnic group, the latest estimates from the 2008 National Health Interview Survey, conducted by the National Center for Health Statistics, smoking rates are 20% for Caucasian women, 24% for Native American women, 18% for African American women, and less than 10% for Asian women.

Women who smoke risk having a heart attack 19 years earlier than nonsmoking women.

The good news is that when you quit smoking, your risk of a heart attack or stroke decreases steadily, approaching that of a nonsmoker in about five years. So it is never too late to quit. Quitting is difficult but possible for everyone. You may need the help and support of your family, physician, and possibly a smoking cessation specialist, so don't hesitate to ask for it. The bottom line is that if you smoke, get help to quit. If someone you love smokes, encourage her to get help to quit.

High Blood Pressure

Having high blood pressure increases the risk for coronary artery disease. *Blood pressure* is the pressure of the blood within the arteries when the heart pumps the blood to the rest of the body. It is measured using an inflatable arm cuff and is referred to in terms of millimeters of mercury (mmHg). During a blood pressure reading, two numbers are measured: systolic blood pressure and diastolic blood pressure. The *systolic blood pressure* is what your pressure is when the heart is contracting, squeezing blood out (during *systole*), and it's the higher number of the reading. The *diastolic pressure* is the pressure when the heart is relaxing (during *diastole*), and it's the lower number of the reading. High blood pressure, known as *hypertension*, is defined as persistent blood pressure that is elevated at or above 140/90 mmHg. Normal blood pressure is defined as blood pressure being less than 120/80 mmHg. The following table outlines the different levels of blood pressure for women, what the levels mean, and how to deal with them.

Categories of Blood Pressure for Adult Women and Treatment Options

Condition	Blood pressure reading	Treatment
Normal	<120/80 mmHg	Prevention of hypertension with healthy lifestyle
Prehypertension	Systolic blood pressure 120–139 mmHg, or diastolic blood pressure 80–89 mmHg	Lifestyle modifications, watchful monitoring
Stage 1 hypertension	Systolic blood pressure 140–159 mmHg, or diastolic blood pressure 90–99 mmHg	Medication, lifestyle modifications
Stage 2 hypertension	Systolic blood pressure ≥160 mmHg, or diastolic blood pressure ≥100 mmHg	Medication, lifestyle modifications

High blood pressure affects the heart in a number of ways. A high pressure system puts excess force on artery walls, and if this continues for too long, it can damage the arteries. A damaged artery is more likely to get plaque buildup over time, resulting in a narrowed artery and reduced blood flow. The arteries to the brain (like the heart arteries) can be affected by high blood pressure, resulting in a stroke. Likewise, the arteries to the kidneys — the *renal arteries* — can be damaged by longstanding hypertension and can cause damage in the kidneys, which can result in complete kidney failure.

Unfortunately, many people have high blood pressure without any symptoms — until it is too late. (If only we had a warning light suggesting we need maintenance, like our cars have!) This is why high blood pressure is known as the silent killer: it comes on silently, potentially causing severe damage without warning. It is for this reason that you need to have your doctor assess your blood pressure at least annually, and more frequently if your blood pressure falls in the prehypertension range or if you have hypertension and have started medication.

Women with hypertension experience a risk of developing coronary artery disease 3.5 times that of females with normal blood pressure. High blood pressure is more common in women taking oral contraceptives, especially in obese women.

When your blood pressure falls outside the normal range, it needs to be monitored closely. Typically, a diagnosis of hypertension is not considered until there have been three separate, elevated readings of your blood pressure. Of course, your blood pressure can be elevated in your doctor's office for several reasons: you may be nervous because you are seeing the doctor (this is known as *white coat hypertension*, when you feel nervous simply from being in a doctor's office); you may have been rushing to get to your appointment (both the emotional and mental stress of being late, and the physical exertion involved may raise your blood pressure); or you may be momentarily stressed or angry. There is also the possibility that your blood pressure reading was taken incorrectly (the cuff and your arm should be at the level of your heart, and the cuff should be right for your arm size).

It is very important for women to know their blood pressure numbers and be aware of what is considered in the normal range. The unfortunate truth is that many women are not well treated when it comes to blood pressure. When a woman's blood pressure is noted to be elevated in a doctor's office, it is less likely to be taken seriously than when the same occurs in a man. Instead, it is often ignored or wrongly attributed to stress or anxiety. So as women, we should ask these questions when getting our blood pressure checked:

♥ What is my blood pressure today?
♥ What should it be?
♥ Is that normal?
♥ Do I need any treatment for this?
♥ When should we recheck this?

Do not allow your high blood pressure to go untreated. Lifestyle changes can lower your blood pressure and many medications are available, if needed. (We discuss medications in greater detail in Chapter 5.) Prehypertension-range blood pressure should be followed closely, since you are at higher risk for developing hypertension. If your doctor is unsure whether your blood pressure is truly elevated and whether the readings in the offices can be relied on, he or she may have you wear an ambulatory blood pressure cuff for 24 hours. It randomly inflates and deflates and will accurately assess your blood pressure outside the doctor's office.

Understanding the language of blood pressure

♥ *Blood pressure* is the force of the blood against the walls of the arteries.

♥ *Hypertension* means high blood pressure.

♥ *Systolic blood pressure* is the highest pressure in the arteries when the heart is pumping blood from the heart to the body.

♥ *Diastolic blood pressure* is the lowest pressure in the arteries when the heart is pumping blood from the heart to the body.

♥ The *brachial artery* is the artery that goes from your shoulder to just below the elbow. It is here that the blood pressure should be measured.

High Cholesterol

High cholesterol is a major risk factor for heart disease. The saturated fats, trans fats, and cholesterol you eat contribute to the cholesterol levels in your blood. Cholesterol is a soft, waxy substance found within the fats that circulate in the bloodstream. It makes sense that if you have too much cholesterol in your bloodstream, you could have more cholesterol deposits, or plaques, in your heart arteries. Cholesterol cannot be absorbed or dissolved in the bloodstream and requires special transporters to remove it from the body. Such transporters are known as lipoproteins, the most important of which are the *low-density lipoprotein* (LDL cholesterol) and the *high-density lipoprotein* (HDL cholesterol).

LDL Cholesterol

LDL cholesterol, or "bad" cholesterol, is the cholesterol that is getting most of the attention these days. When there is too much LDL cholesterol in the bloodstream, it will build up over time on the walls of the arteries of the heart, the brain, and throughout the body, forming plaques that cause narrowing or blockages of the arteries. So a high LDL level — above 160 mg/dL (milligrams per deciliter of blood) or, in metric units, above 4.1 mmol/L (millimole per litre) — is associated with a high risk of heart disease. Nonetheless, an LDL lower than this can still pose a risk for heart disease if other cardiac risk factors are present or if you already have a diagnosis of heart disease. Your target LDL level must be individualized for you, your risk factors, and the presence or absence of certain diseases. If you have heart disease or have had a stroke or suffer from diabetes, your LDL cholesterol should be under 100 mg/dL (<2.6 mmol/L); your doctor may even want it to be under 70 mg/dL (<1.8 mmol/L). The following table outlines the target for LDL cholesterol based on the presence of risk factors for heart disease.

LDL Cholesterol Goals Based on Risk Profile

Current heart disease risk category	LDL goal (mg/dL)
Heart disease or 3 or more risk factors present (10-year risk of heart disease is over 20%)	<100 (<2.6 mmol/L)
2 or more risk factors present (10-year risk of heart disease less than 20%)	<130 (<3.4 mmol/L)
1 or no risk factors present	<160 (<4.1 mmol/L)

Triglycerides

The other component of cholesterol that is routinely measured is triglycerides. Triglycerides also are considered "bad" cholesterol, so the lower your level, the better. Triglycerides circulate in the bloodstream and provide a source of energy. When there are excess triglycerides in circulation, there is an increased risk of a heart attack. This often can occur in people with diabetes or metabolic syndrome. In addition, being overweight or obese, having a poor diet, and being on certain medications can result in very high triglyceride levels. Triglyceride levels should be less than 150 mg/dL (1.7 mmol/L).

HDL Cholesterol

HDL cholesterol, or "good" cholesterol, works to remove cholesterol from the arteries to the liver, which ultimately expels the cholesterol from the body altogether. The higher your level of HDL cholesterol, the better: higher levels appear to reduce the risk of a heart attack. Women with an HDL cholesterol level lower than 50 mg/dL (1.3 mmol/L) are at greater risk for heart disease, regardless of their LDL cholesterol level. This number is higher than what is set for men because it appears that women need to have a higher level of HDL to lower their risk for heart disease.

Cholesterol Breakdown

Cholesterol component	Description	Optimal level for women
Cholesterol*	Combination of *bad* and *good*	<200 mg/dL (<5.2 mmol/L)
HDL	*Good* (think "H" for the higher, the better)	>50 mg/dL (>1.3 mmol/L)
LDL	*Bad* (think "L" for the lower, the better)	<100 mg/dL (<2.6 mmol/L)
Triglycerides	*Bad*	<150 mg/dL (<1.7 mmol/L)
Non-HDL**	*Bad*	30 mg/dL (0.8 mmol/L) more than LDL target

*Total Cholesterol = HDL + LDL + (Triglycerides ÷ 5)
**Non-HDL = Total Cholesterol – HDL

Diabetes

Having diabetes is one of the greatest risk factors for heart disease. In fact, people with diabetes are treated as if they have heart disease because they are at such a high risk for developing it. Diabetes is a disease that results in elevated blood glucose, which can damage the arteries throughout the circulatory system. Damage to the heart arteries and the arteries to the brain increase the risk of heart disease and stroke, respectively. If you have diabetes, you are at least twice as likely to develop cardiovascular disease compared to a non-diabetic. And if you are a woman with diabetes you are at the highest risk for heart disease (three to five times higher risk) compared with a man with diabetes or a non-diabetic man or woman.

> *Women with diabetes have more than double the risk of heart attack than non-diabetic women. Diabetes doubles the risk of a second heart attack in women but not in men. Diabetes affects many more women than men after the age of 45.*

If you are a diabetic, all your cardiac risk factors must be well controlled, and your blood sugar levels must also be well controlled, to reduce the damage to your cardiovascular system. You should be on the same medications as those persons who have heart disease. We discuss this in more detail in Chapter 6.

Physical Inactivity/Poor Physical Fitness

Fitness: If it came in a bottle, everybody would have a great body.
— Cher

Being physically inactive or having a low level of physical fitness is another major risk factor for heart disease. Physical activity reduces the impact and presence of other cardiac risk factors. It improves and maintains your fitness level, and it improves cholesterol, blood pressure, and diabetes. Being physically active also helps weight control and has so many other benefits for the whole body. It is estimated that at least 35% of deaths due to cardiovascular disease are because of physical inactivity. This number is quite remarkable, and given that only about 20% of the U.S. population reports getting regular physical activity for 30 minutes a day at least five days a week, this is a highly prevalent risk factor. Physical inactivity is more prevalent in women than in men, so this is a risk factor that we need to address.

Metabolic Syndrome

Metabolic syndrome is a risk factor for heart disease. The syndrome consists of a cluster of risk factors that are associated with insulin resistance and identified by central, or abdominal, obesity — the "apple shape" (as compared to a "pear shape") when it comes to body types. You may have a normal weight yet still have an abnormal waist circumference, and waist circumference is a better predictor of your risk of heart disease than weight or body mass index. For women, central obesity is described as a waist circumference greater than 35 inches (88 centimeters), but this number can vary depending on race or ethnicity and which definitions of waist circumference are used (see the table on the next page).

The syndrome's cluster of risk factors are central obesity, elevated blood sugar, systolic blood pressure over 135 mmHg or diastolic blood pressure over 85 mmHg, low HDL (under 50 mg/dL), and triglycerides greater than 150 mg/dL. If you have three or more of these risk factors, you have metabolic syndrome. And this cluster of risk factors is associated with an increased risk of developing both diabetes and heart disease. Metabolic syndrome is increasing in the U.S. population, with more than 25% of all women having the metabolic syndrome.

Having a waist circumference above 35 inches or 88 centimeters (cm) is abnormal for any group, but maximum acceptable waist measurements may be smaller than that. We list the more precise numbers of waist circumference by ethnic background in the table below. Note that your waist size is not your pant size. Rather, waist circumference is measured along the top of the iliac crests (the prominent bone you can feel when you put your hands to your sides, just below your waist) and across the belly button.

High-Risk Waist Circumference for Women, by Race and Ethnicity

Group	Circumference
Caucasian	>35 inches (88 cm)
African descent	>35 inches (88 cm)
Central and South American	>31.5 inches (80 cm)
South Asian	>31.5 inches (80 cm)
Chinese	>31.5 inches (80 cm)
Japanese	>35.5 inches (90 cm)
Middle Eastern, Mediterranean	>31.5 inches (80 cm)

Obesity

Obesity is a risk factor for heart disease and an obesity epidemic is a worldwide concern as rates in children and adults are increasing everywhere. Obesity is defined by a measure known as body mass index (BMI). It is the ratio of weight to height squared, measured in kilograms per square meter (kg/m^2). Think of it like your weight proportionate to your body size. A normal BMI is less than 25 kg/m^2. If you have a BMI of 25 to 29.9 kg/m^2, you are considered to be overweight. And obesity is defined as a BMI greater than 30 kg/m^2. So if you are overweight or obese, you may say you are too short for your weight. Unfortunately, as adults, we can't grow in height, so the only thing we can change is our weight. Currently in the United States and Canada, approximately two out of every three people are either overweight or obese and this number appears to be increasing annually.

It may be obvious why being obese is associated with heart disease. For instance, obesity is associated with many of the other cardiac risk factors we've discussed: a person who is obese is more likely to have high blood pressure, diabetes, metabolic syndrome, and abnormal cholesterol (particularly low HDL and elevated triglycerides). Having excess body weight is also associated with increased inflammation, which may increase the risk for heart disease. Obesity can also result in inactivity, which can only increase the risk further. The greater your weight, the greater your risk for heart disease.

So if you know your BMI, discuss it and your weight with your doctor. If weight is a risk factor for you, know that you can change it.

Stress, Depression, and Anxiety

Stress, depression, and anxiety are most definitely risk factors for heart disease. Stress can be difficult to define and measure, and it may affect one person differently than it does another. Among other causes, stress can be a result of a job, social isolation, emotional events, or mental tension. Chronic stress can affect other risk factors for heart disease: it can increase blood pressure, damage the heart arteries, and increase inflammation and coagulation. It is also associated with irregular heart rhythms. As well, stress can result in high-risk behaviors that can adversely affect the heart like overeating, physical inactivity, not getting enough sleep, and smoking. It is important to recognize that stress can affect your heart and to know that if you are under a lot of stress — and particularly if you are not dealing with that stress well — you should discuss this with your doctor. Ignoring your stress can affect your heart, particularly if it goes on for a long time.

> *Negative emotions and depression are risk factors for heart attack and stroke. Conversely, happier people are less likely to develop heart disease.*

Like stress, both depression and anxiety can increase the risk of a heart attack. If someone who has had a heart attack or stroke has depression, that person has a higher risk of suffering a subsequent heart attack. Untreated depression in someone who has undergone coronary artery bypass surgery is associated with a greater risk of death. And it is not uncommon for someone to have depression after a heart attack, stroke, or coronary artery bypass surgery. But doctors, concentrating on issues related to the patient's cardiovascular system, sometimes forget to ask about it. So be sure to bring it up if you're feeling depressed and your doctor has not raised the issue. Don't let depression go untreated. It is important to recognize the close relationship between the mind and the heart and to take care of both. In Chapter 10 we discuss stress in further detail — how it affects women and our hearts and what you can do to better manage stress.

> People who live alone are twice as likely to have a heart attack or sudden cardiac death as those who live with a partner or roommate.

Sleep Apnea

Sleep apnea is a chronic condition that disrupts sleep. It is quite common, affecting about one in every 50 women. But you may be surprised to hear that if you suffer from sleep apnea, you are at greater risk for heart disease. Sleep apnea is a condition where you stop breathing, for seconds or even minutes, multiple times during sleep, blocking airflow to the lungs. This affects your deep sleep period and is one of the reasons for waking up fatigued after what should have been a good night's rest. When this occurs repeatedly for a long period, the chronic reduction in oxygen to the blood can adversely affect blood vessels in the heart and lungs, resulting in high blood pressure, pulmonary hypertension, heart failure, *atrial fibrillation* (a common type of heart arrhythmia), and coronary artery disease. The most common type of sleep apnea is obstructive sleep apnea, where the upper airway around the neck is blocked. The condition is more common in people who are overweight or obese but being overweight or obese is not the only cause of sleep apnea.

So, if you wake up fatigued despite sleeping what should be long enough, if you snore, and if you find yourself dropping off to sleep during the day, you should be assessed for sleep apnea. Treating sleep apnea can reduce the risk of having heart problems in the future.

Sleep

Sleep is a modifiable risk factor for heart disease development, as recent studies have shown. Getting too little sleep puts you at a higher risk for developing heart disease, but getting too much sleep may also adversely affect your heart. A study of over 30,000 American adults published in 2010 found that the optimal amount of sleep appears to be seven hours.[1] Sleep time was calculated as the total time of sleep (including naps) in a 24-hour period. The researchers found that those who slept five hours or less a day had twice the risk of having angina, coronary heart disease, a heart attack, or a stroke. Similarly, those who slept more than nine hours a day were one and a half times more likely to develop cardiovascular disease. The risk to the heart and vascular system from lack of sleep was particularly strong in those 60 years or younger and in women. Women who got too little sleep (five hours or less) were at the highest risk of developing heart disease or having a stroke — about two and a half times greater the risk than women who got seven hours of sleep.

The exact ways in which sleep, whether too much or too little, can affect the heart and vascular system are not clear. However, certainly sleep affects the metabolism and endocrine systems of the body. Too little sleep has been shown to adversely affect glucose metabolism and insulin sensitivity and it can cause weight gain and raise blood pressure, all of which may affect the heart and contribute to the development of cardiovascular disease.

Just as too little or too much of anything can be bad for us, we all need sleep, but in moderation. The American Academy of Sleep Medicine recommends that adults get about seven to eight hours of sleep a night.

Emerging Risk Factors
High-Sensitivity C-Reactive Protein

High-sensitivity C-reactive protein (hs-CRP), a protein found in the blood that is measured in milligrams per liter (mg/L), is the risk marker making news these days. Should everyone have this protein checked? Is there a treatment for an elevated hs-CRP? Does an elevated hs-CRP by itself warrant treatment with *statins* (the class of drugs often used to lower cholesterol levels — see Chapter 5 for more about statins)? The debate rages on and on.

Certainly hs-CRP is a risk marker for heart disease, meaning an elevation in hs-CRP is associated with the development of heart disease. It appears to be a marker of inflammation and can fluctuate — for instance, if you have an infection or inflammation when your blood work is done, it is likely that your hs-CRP may be elevated because of this infection or inflammation. Once the infection or inflammation is gone, your hs-CRP may be lower. But if your hs-CRP is elevated in your usual state of health, it may be a marker of increased inflammation within the vascular system. And this might be important for the heart, as we have known for years that inflammation is part of the process that causes coronary artery disease, possibly triggering a heart attack.

That hs-CRP is elevated in those who develop heart disease is important. But what is still not clear is where this risk marker is a risk mediator. That is, if we lower the level of hs-CRP, can we lower the risk of heart disease? Should therapy be based on hs-CRP alone? The answer remains obscure. Recently, an important study, the JUPITER Study, released its findings.[2] The study took people with a normal LDL level but an elevated hs-CRP (above 2.0 mg/L) and randomized the participants to either get a statin medication called rosuvastatin or a placebo. By current guidelines, this group of people would normally not be treated with a statin. What the study found was that those who got the medication did better over time. They had a 44% reduction in cumulative risk for a heart attack, stroke, need for cardiac surgery or artery stenting, hospitalization for angina, and death. But the findings did not prove that checking hs-CRP had a causal role in the development of cardiovascular disease or that it was a useful marker to check in everyone to dictate treatment. As well, those in the study who were given the statin medication had a greater likelihood of developing diabetes. There are concerns, too, regarding how low an LDL can safely be, because LDL will fall when a statin is used. So it is controversial whether hs-CRP should be checked, if it is helpful to check it, and what to do if hs-CRP levels are high. In our opinion, if it will not change your treatment, then it shouldn't be checked. If the results will help you and your doctor determine your risk and treatment, then check it. Discuss with your doctor what's right for you.

Apolipoprotein B

Apolipoprotein B (ApoB) is part of the composition of LDL cholesterol and triglycerides. It is not yet routinely measured when cholesterol is checked but is thought to be an even better predictor of the risk for cardiovascular disease than LDL cholesterol. ApoB attaches itself to receptors on cells to draw cholesterol into those cells. A high ApoB level is associated with plaque formation, which results in cardiovascular disease. The level of ApoB may be elevated because of poor diet, genetic reasons, or a combination of both. Also, some ApoB genetic abnormalities can result in a much higher risk for premature cardiovascular disease. It is not standard to check ApoB, although some guidelines, including those of the American Diabetes Association and the American College of Cardiology, are suggesting that ApoB or LDL cholesterol can be used to assess risk and have published targeted levels of ApoB to achieve, based on risk factors.[3] At some point, it will likely become commonplace to check ApoB, given its strength at predicting cardiovascular disease, so discuss with your doctor if you should have this checked. The following table outlines target LDL cholesterol and ApoB levels that high risk women should be at based on cardiovascular risk factors.

LDL and ApoB Goals for High-Risk Patients

Risk group	Description	LDL target	ApoB target
High risk	No diabetes or heart disease, but >2 cardiac risk factors present Diabetes without any other risk factors	<100 mg/dL (<2.6 mmol/L)	<90 mg/dL (<2.3 mmol/L)
Highest risk	Known cardiovascular disease Diabetes with >1 cardiac risk factors	<70 mg/dL (<1.8 mmol/L)	<80 mg/dL (<2.1 mmol/L)

Lipoprotein(a)

Lipoprotein(a), or Lp(a), is a genetic variation of LDL. Having a high level of Lp(a) may be associated with a greater risk of developing heart disease prematurely. But how exactly Lp(a) increases the risk is not clear, though it is thought that it may accelerate the buildup of fatty deposits along the arteries. Lp(a) is also *prothrombotic*, meaning it increases the ability of blood clots to form. Lp(a) levels have the greatest hereditary link of all emerging risk markers and are also related to race — often being higher in Caucasians and Asians. There is no established treatment for an elevated Lp(a) and not all studies show a relationship between an elevated Lp(a) and heart disease. For this reason, Lp(a) is not routinely checked when screening for cardiovascular risk factors.

Homocysteine

Another risk marker for heart disease is homocysteine. Homocysteine is an amino acid found in the blood and its increased levels are associated with cardiovascular disease (heart disease and stroke), particularly when other cardiac risk factors are present. There are plausible theories for how homocysteine may increase cardiovascular risk: it may promote injury of blood vessels, alter platelet activity, inhibit dilation of blood vessels, and even cause increased blood clots. Some genetic abnormalities are associated with particularly high homocystcine levels.

It had been thought that treating high homocysteine levels with folic acid would reduce cardiovascular risk, because increasing folic acid intake reduces homocysteine levels. But multiple trials in the past few years have shown that using folic acid supplements does not reduce the development or recurrence of cardiovascular disease and, in fact, the potential for harm may actually increase by using them. Taking folic acid supplements in an attempt to reduce heart disease risk is not recommended. (Of course, if you are pregnant, it's important to take folic acid to protect your developing baby.) Rather, the American Heart Association recommends eating foods rich in folate (the naturally occurring form of folic acid), such as fruits and green leafy vegetables. And as for checking your homocysteine levels? At this time it is not suggested to routinely check these levels, as no recommended treatment exists for high levels.

Fibrinogen

Fibrinogen is a protein in the blood that promotes blood clotting when there is vascular or tissue injury. Fibrinogen is necessary in normal amounts, but when levels are excessively high, it may cause unnecessary blood clots. For this reason elevated fibrinogen levels are associated with cardiovascular disease. Currently, there are no therapies to lower fibrinogen level, so this is only a marker for cardiovascular disease and should not be checked routinely.

Lipoprotein Subfractions

Lipoprotein subfractions are emerging as useful markers for better heart disease risk assessment. Many properties of lipoproteins are not apparent by simply reporting the LDL, HDL, and triglycerides. Lipoproteins have different sizes and densities, and the measured concentrations of LDL and HDL represent not just one lipoprotein but a spectrum of their particles of different sizes and densities. Small LDL particles appear to increase risk for cardiovascular disease more than large LDL particles do. Conversely, larger HDL particles are more protective than smaller HDL particles. Oxidized LDL, which is a more dangerous LDL form, increases the risk for cardiovascular disease. So lipoprotein quality may matter more than quantity, and can be detected by assessing lipoprotein subfractions. Certain medications have been shown to alter particle size.

But what is not clear is whether targeting these subfractions is more effective at reducing cardiovascular risk compared with testing cholesterol levels alone. Lipoprotein subfractions are not routinely assessed, but doing so can be useful to determine a person's response to therapy. Also, assessing lipoprotein subfractions may be useful for women with no cardiac risk factors other than a family history of premature coronary artery disease, with a normal cholesterol panel.

The Heart of the Matter

Ultimately, to determine the risk of developing heart disease, you need to consider the risk factors that apply to you, as well as the risk factors that do not apply to you. Knowing this information is the first step toward reducing your risk. So make sure your risk factors are routinely assessed and understand that they can change over time, so see your doctor regularly. Know your numbers, ask for all your numbers, and if your numbers are not on target but you're not getting treatment, make sure you know why. If you are getting treatment, make sure that your progress and treatment are monitored over time. Knowledge is powerful, so be empowered to use what you know about your modifiable risk factors to work with your doctor and direct your own heart care for the best protection possible.

Chapter 3

Determining Your Risk of Heart Disease

Living at risk is jumping off the cliff and building your wings on the way down.
— Ray Bradbury

By now you are aware of what puts you at risk for heart disease. So let's look at how you can assess your own risk of developing heart disease and, if you have risk factors, determine your odds of developing heart disease in the short term (in the next 10 years), as well as in your lifetime.

Indeed, physicians have been shifting their way of thinking about risk assessment in women. Over the years, many women have been left with the perception that they are at very low risk of developing heart disease because they are young and calculate only their 10-year risk. However, not only is periodically recalculating the short-term risk useful, but doing so helps to assess your lifetime risk. Knowing your odds of developing heart disease can help you see what factors you can change to reduce your risk and can guide your therapy and treatment based on your risk assessment. After all, being at risk does not mean you will definitely get heart disease; knowing your risk is your first line of defense against heart disease.

Risk Classifications

There are essentially three categories of heart disease risk for women:
High Risk, At Risk, and Optimal Risk.[1] Every woman fits into one of
these categories. The following table defines each category:

Cardiovascular Disease Risk Categories

Risk category	Criteria
High Risk	Established heart disease
	Cerebrovascular disease (stroke, carotid disease)
	Peripheral arterial disease (PAD)
	Abdominal aortic aneurysm
	End-stage or chronic kidney disease
	Diabetes
	10-year Framingham Risk* >20%
At Risk	One or more major risk factors for cardiovascular disease, including:
	Cigarette smoking
	Poor diet
	Physical inactivity
	Obesity, central obesity (waist circumference of >35 inches/ 88 cm)
	Family history of early heart disease (heart disease at under 65 years of age in female relative and under 55 years of age in male relative)
	Hypertension
	High cholesterol
	Evidence of subclinical vascular disease (coronary calcification)
	Metabolic syndrome
	Poor fitness on treadmill test and/or abnormal heart rate recovery
Optimal Risk	10-year Framingham Risk* <10% and a healthy lifestyle, with no risk factors

* See the "Short-Term Risk" section below for a discussion of the Framingham Risk Score.

If you look at these categories, you will see that only a woman with absolutely no risk factors and a healthy lifestyle can be in the Optimal Risk category. The majority of people fall into either the High Risk or At Risk group.

> *Every year 435,000 American women have heart attacks. Of these women, 83,000 are under age 65 and 35,000 are under age 55. Their average age is 70.4.*

Regardless of which category a woman falls into, based on the American Heart Association's *Evidence-Based Guidelines for Cardiovascular Disease Prevention in Women,* all women are recommended to incorporate therapeutic lifestyle changes to improve their cardiovascular health, such as those we suggest in the box below.

Therapeutic lifestyle changes

♥ Smoking cessation

♥ Heart-healthy eating

♥ Regular physical activity (60 to 90 minutes of moderate to intense physical activity on most, and preferably all, days of the week)

♥ Weight maintenance

Everyone, regardless of risk category, will benefit from incorporating or continuing these proven therapeutic lifestyle changes, which we discuss more in later chapters.

Based on these same guidelines, women considered to be High Risk require treatment with aggressive goals — particularly in terms of cholesterol and targeting lower LDL. At Risk women should have individual risk factors treated as recommended in Chapter 2 to lower their short-term risk and reduce their lifetime risk of developing heart disease.

So determining which category — High Risk, At Risk, or Optimal Risk — you fall into is one way of quickly assessing your risk. But two other types of assessment are important to put your own heart disease risk assessment together: short-term and long-term risk.

Short-Term Risk

Short-term risk is best assessed using the Framingham Risk Score, a tool recommended by both the American Heart Association's *Evidence-Based Guidelines for Cardiovascular Disease Prevention in Women* and the National Cholesterol Education Program's *Adult Treatment Panel III* (ATP III). The Reynolds Risk Score is also a reasonable tool to use for short-term risk assessment, but it needs more validation before it can be recommended over the Framingham Risk Score. It is less widely accepted because it requires that hs-CRP be measured, which, as we noted in Chapter 2, is currently not recommended. There are other reasonable tools that are used in Europe, including the United Kingdom, but the most widely accepted and the basis of most American and Canadian guidelines is the Framingham Risk Score.

The Framingham Risk Score is a formulated score giving a certain "weight" to the presence or absence of risk factors. This score was developed from the Framingham Heart Study, which followed both men and women in the Massachusetts city of Framingham. The study began in 1948 to measure risk factors for heart disease, monitoring this population for heart disease development over time. The study is ongoing and has been supported by the National Institutes of Health.

In the first year after a heart attack, women are more than 50% more likely to die than men are. In the first six years after a heart attack, women are almost twice as likely to have a second heart attack.

Based on the cohort of women from the Framingham Heart Study, the risk factors that appear to matter the most for heart disease development and that are used to calculate the risk are gender, age, total cholesterol level, HDL cholesterol level, blood pressure, and smoking. *The higher your Framingham Risk Score, the greater your risk of developing heart disease or dying from heart disease in the next 10 years.* Low risk is a Framingham Risk Score of 19 or less, where the odds of developing heart disease in the next 10 years are less than 10%. Intermediate risk is a score of 20 to 22, where the odds of developing heart disease in the next 10 years are between 10 and 20%. High risk is a score above 22 — or having heart disease or diabetes or any other factor listed in the High Risk category (see the "Cardiovascular Disease Risk Categories" table earlier in this chapter) where the odds of developing heart disease are greater than 20%. You can calculate your Framingham Risk Score using the charts below, if you know your numbers.

Calculating Your Framingham Risk Score to Assess Your 10-Year Risk of Heart Disease

Step 1: Calculate score for <u>Age</u>

Age	Points
20–34	-7
35–39	-3
40–44	0
45–49	3
50–54	6
55–59	8
60–64	10
65–69	12
70–74	14

Step 2: Calculate score for <u>Cholesterol</u> by age (based on mg/dL*)

Total Cholesterol	Age 20–39	Age 40–49	Age 50–59	Age 60–69	Age 70–79
<160	0	0	0	0	0
160–199	4	3	2	1	1
200–239	8	6	4	2	1
240–279	11	8	5	3	2
280+	13	10	7	4	2

*To convert from metric units (mmol/L) to mg/dL, multiply by 0.0259

Step 3: Calculate score for <u>Smoking</u> by age

	Age 20–39	Age 40–49	Age 50–59	Age 60–69	Age 70–79
Nonsmoker	0	0	0	0	0
Smoker	9	7	4	2	1

Step 4: Calculate score for <u>HDL</u> (based on mg/dL*)

HDL	Points
60+	-1
50–59	0
40–49	1
<40	2

*To convert from metric units (mmol/L) to mg/dL, multiply by 0.0259

Step 5: Calculate score for <u>Systolic Blood Pressure</u> if treated or untreated

Systolic BP	Untreated	Treated
<120	0	0
120–129	1	3
130–139	2	4
140–159	3	5
160+	4	6

Step 6: Add up points to get Framingham Risk Score (10-Year Risk for Heart Disease)

Total points	10–year risk
Low	
<9	<1%
9	1%
10	1%
11	1%
12	1%
13	2%
14	2%
15	3%
16	4%
17	5%
18	6%
19	8%
Intermediate	
20	11%
21	14%
22	17%
High	
23	22%
24	27%
25 or more	>30%

Source: National Heart, Lung, and Blood Institute; National Institutes of Health; U.S. Department of Health and Human Services

Lifetime Risk

As I see it, every day you do one of two things: build health or produce disease in yourself.

— Adelle Davis

Of course, your 10-year risk for heart disease tells you only your risk in the next 10 years. But over those 10 years, things can change. Certainly, we all get older, our lifestyles can change, and our risk factors may change no matter what adjustments we make to our activity levels or diets.

This is why it's important to also calculate your lifetime risk: we have come to appreciate that the 10-year assessment is just not enough. The majority of women (over 80%) will be placed as low risk by the 10-year risk score, but about two out of three women in this low risk group have a higher risk of developing cardiovascular disease in their lifetime.

A very good tool exists to estimate lifetime risk. It is based on the Framingham Heart Study and was developed by researchers at Chicago's Northwestern University. This tool shows that if at the age of 50 you have no traditional cardiac risk factors present, your lifetime risk of developing cardiovascular disease is very low and you are more likely to live longer, compared with women with any cardiac risk factors present.[2] We know that one in every three women will develop heart disease in her lifetime. But this risk is obviously lower for women without any cardiac risk factors. So the ideal goal is to prevent any modifiable risk factors from occurring and treating the ones you have.

Use the chart below to assess your lifetime risk. If you are under the age of 50 but have cardiac risk factors already present, your risk of developing heart disease is already higher than those without traditional cardiac risk factors present, regardless of age. Once you turn 50, you look at the presence or absence of traditional risk factors to estimate your lifetime risk.

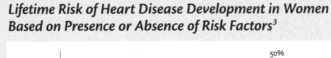

Lifetime Risk of Heart Disease Development in Women Based on Presence or Absence of Risk Factors[3]

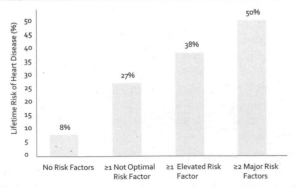

Optimal risk factors =   *untreated total cholesterol <180 mg/dL*
(<4.65 mmol/L)

+

untreated blood pressure <120/<80 mmHg

+

nonsmoker

+

no diabetes

Not optimal risk factors =   *untreated total cholesterol 180 to 199 mg/*
dL (4.65 to 5.15 mmol/L), OR

untreated systolic blood pressure 120 to
139 mmHg or diastolic blood pressure 80
to 89 mmHg,

+

nonsmoker

+

no diabetes

Elevated risk factors =   *untreated total cholesterol 200 to*
*239 mg/dL (5.16 to 6.19 mmol/L), **OR***
untreated systolic blood pressure 140
to 159 mmHg or diastolic blood pressure
90 to 99 mmHg,

+

nonsmoker

+

no diabetes

Major risk factors =   *total cholesterol >240 mg/dL (>6.20*
*mmol/L) or treated high cholesterol, **OR***
systolic blood pressure >160 mmHg,
diastolic blood pressure >100 mmHg, or
treated high blood pressure, OR
smoker, OR
diabetes

As you can see, this estimation tool relies on the presence or absence of risk factors. By estimating your lifetime risk and seeing long-term impact of your risk factors on your heart, you are better able to address and minimize these risk factors.

The Heart of the Matter

A woman is the full circle. Within her is the power to create, nurture, and transform.

— Diane Mariechild

Ultimately, your risk of developing heart disease comes down to whether you have risk factors present. Of course, some risk factors can't be avoided, but they do need to be controlled. If you are aware of your risk factors at a young age, you can work to prevent the modifiable ones from developing and to attain the best control possible of any non-modifiable ones. But knowing your risks at any point in your life enables you to put into motion the changes necessary to save your heart and save your life.

Chapter 4

Screening and Testing for Heart Disease: What Must Be Done, What Can Be Done, and What the Results Mean

The only way to pass a test is to take the test.
— Marlo Morgan

In Chapters 2 and 3, we emphasized the importance of being screened for heart disease to know your risk and know your risk factors. There are numerous tests that your doctor can order to screen for heart disease. There are some tests that every woman should have done as part of a routine health check, while other tests are done only because of a physical finding in an exam, specific symptoms you are experiencing, or an abnormal result in an earlier test. Discuss with your doctor which tests are suitable for you. It is important that you understand what the tests are and why they are being done, what the tests can — and cannot — reveal about your heart, and what the test results mean. It is also important to know the risks of any test before undergoing it.

Most tests are *noninvasive*, meaning that no instruments — other than perhaps a needle to draw blood or a catheter to access a vein — are inserted into the body and there is no cutting or incision made into the body. The risks of such tests are much lower than *invasive* tests, where instruments *are* inserted into the body. In this chapter, we take a look at the tests that commonly screen for heart disease or its risk factors. We'll tell you who should get them, what their purposes are, and what risks they may involve.

Noninvasive Tests

As we mentioned, noninvasive tests do not involve any instruments being inserted into the body, except perhaps a needle to get blood or a catheter to access a vein.

Cholesterol/Lipid Evaluation

Method: Blood is drawn after a person has been fasting for 10 to 12 hours.

Purpose: A woman's blood cholesterol levels should be checked at age 20 and then repeated as often as needed based on baseline levels, treatment and medication changes, lifestyle changes, weight gain, and family history, in addition to clinical findings that suggest high cholesterol (for example, skin eruptions).

Results: See the tables on cholesterol goals on page 30 for more on what your numbers mean.

Risks: There is some risk of bleeding and bruising at the site of blood draw (where the needle is inserted).

Cardiac Enzymes (Cardiac Biomarkers)

Method: Blood is drawn but no fasting is required.

Purpose: Cardiac enzymes or biomarkers will be drawn if you have symptoms or electrocardiogram (ECG) abnormalities that suggest you may have angina or an ongoing heart attack. This test is often done in the emergency room or doctor's office when a person has signs and symptoms that are consistent with a reduction of blood flow to the heart (*ischemia*). Typically, the levels of the cardiac enzymes *troponin* or *creatine kinase-MB* (CK-MB, which is an isoenzyme of the enzyme creatine kinase), or both, are checked. These enzymes, when elevated, usually reflect damage to the heart muscle. Troponin is more specific than creatine kinase (CK-MB) for heart damage. Usually two to three levels of cardiac enzymes are measured over a 12- to 16-hour period, depending on hospital protocol.

Results: Normally, troponin levels are undetectable unless there is some heart damage, and troponin levels can remain elevated for one to two weeks after a heart attack. It is true that troponin may be elevated with strenuous exercise, but this elevation is generally not a concern if a person has no other symptoms of heart damage. CK-MB levels can also be elevated if there is skeletal muscle damage. Clinical assessment of symptoms and signs will ultimately determine whether follow-up or treatment is needed for abnormal or even normal levels of troponin and CK-MB.

Risks: Risk exists of bleeding and bruising at the site of blood draw (where the needle is inserted).

Blood Glucose
Method: Blood is drawn after fasting for at least eight hours.

Purpose: This test can screen for diabetes by measuring the sugar levels in the blood after a period of fasting. If you have already been diagnosed with diabetes, your blood glucose will be tested routinely as part of your diabetes control. As 65% of diabetics die from heart disease and stroke, it is obvious that avoiding the disease altogether is preferable. But if you do have diabetes, you can reduce your risk of a heart attack or stroke by making sure your diabetes is well controlled.

Results: At a certain level of fasting blood glucose, the diagnosis of diabetes is automatically made. (You'll find normal and abnormal levels of glucose listed in the table below.) Although the test is often part of routine blood tests, screening blood glucose levels is essential for people with a family history of diabetes, those who are overweight, those over the age of 40, and women who are pregnant. If you are pregnant, the thresholds for fasting glucose are higher than what is considered normal for non-pregnant women. Women diagnosed with gestational diabetes are at high risk of developing diabetes in the future, even many years after a pregnancy, so their fasting blood glucose should be routinely checked to screen for this.

Fasting Glucose Levels

	U.S. Guidelines	Canadian Guidelines
Normal	70–99 mg/dL	<6.1 mmol/L
Glucose intolerance	100–125 mg/dL	6.1–6.9 mmol/L
Diabetic	>125 mg/dL	≥7.0 mmol/L

Risks: A potential risk is bleeding and bruising at the site of blood draw (where the needle is inserted).

Hemoglobin A1c

Method: Blood drawn and no fasting is required.

Purpose: *Glycosylated hemoglobin A1c* (HbA1c) is used to assess diabetes control over the past three months. In contrast, a fasting blood glucose really only reflects the previous 24 hours or less. HbA1c can also be used to screen or diagnose diabetes. Those with chronic kidney or liver disease, anemia or recent bleeding or recent blood transfusions, and pregnant women should not take this test.

Results: HbA1c is reported as a percentage, which can be calculated into an average blood glucose level.

HbA1c Results Interpretation

	HbA1c Level
Normal	4–6%
Prediabetes	5.7–6.4%
Diabetes	>6.5%
Diabetes control target	<7%

Risks: There is a risk of bleeding and bruising at the site of blood draw (where the needle is inserted).

Electrocardiogram (ECG)

Method: To perform an *electrocardiogram*, painless electrodes are applied to the chest to measure the heart's electrical activity. Typically, a 12-lead ECG is performed, where 12 electrical signals are recorded at roughly the same time, using a total of 10 electrodes attached to the chest. The electrodes are combined into pairs to make up a *lead*, which is the output from each pair.

Purpose: An ECG may be performed for several reasons. It might be done based on symptoms to assess for a heart attack, or it might be done during stress testing to check for reduced blood flow to the heart. It can also be done if there is an abnormal heart rhythm during a physical exam or if you are experiencing palpitations, as the ECG can reveal if there is an irregular heart rhythm (*arrhythmia*).

Results: ECG results can diagnose a heart attack (whether new or old), ischemia, heart conduction abnormalities, heart rate assessment, arrhythmias, blood clots that have gone to the lungs (*pulmonary embolisms*), and fluid around the heart (*pericardial effusions* and *tamponade*), in addition to other abnormalities in the heart. There is no one straightforward way of interpreting an ECG tracing; rather, there are typical normal features, some variants of normal, and many abnormalities that may require further testing if they show up.

Risks: None.

Research suggests that 25% of heart attacks go unrecognized and are discovered only later when a routine ECG is performed.

Signal Average Electrocardiogram

Method: A *signal average electrocardiogram* (SAECG) is an ECG with special software that computes an average of the heart's contraction activity. In contrast to the regular ECG, which takes seconds to perform, a SAECG takes from 7 to 10 minutes to record this information.

Purpose: The SAECG is not commonly used anymore but can be ordered to assess for arrhythmias from the ventricle, particularly after a heart attack.

Results: The abnormality assessed on a SAECG is a variation in the late ventricular potentials, which means that there is a difference in the electrical signal of the heart in the latter part of the heart's contraction. Identifying this difference indicates who is at high risk for sudden cardiac death or other ventricular arrhythmias.

Risks: None.

Echocardiogram

Method: An *echocardiogram*, often referred to as an echo, is a *sonogram* — an ultrasound image of the interior of the heart, created through the use of sound waves. A probe, which emits sound waves, is held to the chest directly over the heart; when the sound waves make contact with solid structures in the heart, such as chambers and valves, they send sound waves back to the probe that are used to construct a moving image of the heart. Images are usually two-dimensional, unless three-dimensional (3-D) technology is specifically used. There are three main types of echocardiograms:

♥ *Transthoracic echocardiogram (TTE):* This type is the most common echocardiogram. Gel is applied to the chest and to the ultrasound probe, which is then placed on the chest. The probe is moved around to get images of the whole heart. This noninvasive test is highly accurate if good images are produced. It generally takes about 30 minutes for a full examination, unless abnormalities are noted, in which case the doctor or technician may spend more time to capture further images.

♥ *Transesophageal echocardiogram (TEE):* This type is specifically used when particular parts of the heart require a better view than what would be captured using other types of echocardiograms. A probe with an ultrasound tip is inserted through the mouth and down the esophagus. For this reason, the patient is sedated with medication. Although TEEs are more invasive than transthoracic echocardiograms, they are quite routine and generally well tolerated. The test typically takes about an hour.

♥ *Three-dimensional echocardiogram:* A 3-D echocardiography can be part of any type of echocardiogram but is used specifically to better show issues with heart valves and some types of heart defects, which are better viewed using 3-D images. Surgeons may want a 3-D image of the heart before or during surgery to better view the heart problem. Since developing 3-D images takes more time, this test is done only when needed.

Below is an image of a transthoracic echocardiogram, with the ultrasound probe placed on the chest wall close to the ventricles (top of the image), resulting in what looks like an "upside down" appearance of the heart with the ventricles on top and the atria on the bottom. This is how your cardiologist will view your heart using a transthoracic echocardiogram. Pictured is how a normal heart appears.

Transthoracic Echocardiogram Image

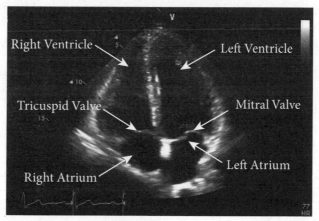

Courtesy of Dr. Priya Kohli, MD, Northwestern University

Purpose: An echocardiogram is usually ordered to check for and evaluate the following conditions:
- ♥ heart murmur
- ♥ heart damage after a heart attack
- ♥ heart function (*myocardium*) if symptoms suggest damage to the heart or if there are symptoms of heart failure
- ♥ heart function if there is concern that the heartbeat is irregular (*arrhythmia*)
- ♥ the pericardium surrounding the heart
- ♥ infection of the heart valves (*endocarditis*)

Results: A cardiologist will examine the echocardiographic images (either while the test is being done or at a later time) and comment on anything that is not normal, even on mild abnormalities or variants of normal. Even insignificant findings that have no health implications will be commented on in an echo report. Nonetheless, the purpose of an echocardiogram is to identify structural abnormalities of the heart and any abnormalities in its functioning. Images of surrounding structures of the heart may also be captured and commented on if abnormalities are seen.

We recommend that if you are having an echocardiogram, you get it done at an accredited echo laboratory, so that you can be confident that the images and interpretations are reliable. In the United States and Canada, these echo laboratories are certified by the Intersocietal Commission for the Accreditation of Echocardiography Laboratories (ICAEL). In the United Kingdom, the accreditation comes from the British Society of Echocardiography. In Europe, such laboratories will be accredited by the European Association of Echocardiography (EAE).

Risks: No known risks or side effects.

Exercise Stress Test

Method: In an exercise stress test, you will be required to exercise, either on a treadmill or bicycle, while your heart rate and blood pressure are monitored, sometimes with imaging on an ECG machine or even with nuclear imaging. You will also be monitored for symptoms and fatigue. In most cases, this test is a *symptom-limited* stress test, meaning that your symptoms will determine when you stop. When to stop the test is up to the judgment of the supervising physician, who may end the test even if you are not showing any symptoms but he or she sees something concerning or dangerous occurring on the ECG or with your vital signs. For example, it is abnormal if blood pressure does not rise and very abnormal if the blood pressure drops. Heart rate is expected to rise, unless you are on medication that prevents this. Dangerous arrhythmias can occur with stress testing and may be a sign of reduced blood flow to the heart — the ECG monitors for this risk.

In another type of exercise stress test, you will be asked to wear a face mask while your oxygen to carbon monoxide level is measured. This is commonly done on persons with heart failure to assess whether they are candidates for a heart transplant, but it may also be done on persons with pulmonary hypertension.

Purpose: The following are reasons that you might undergo exercise stress testing:
- ♥ to assess for coronary heart disease, usually due to symptoms of chest pressure, chest pain, shortness of breath with exertion, or any

symptoms that make your doctor concerned about reduced blood flow to the heart muscle

♥ to assess coronary artery disease based on an abnormality on an ECG

♥ to see if you are physically able to begin an exercise program, particularly if you are fairly sedentary

♥ to test the effectiveness of any procedure (coronary artery bypass surgery or a coronary artery stent or angioplasty) that has been done to improve blood flow to the heart

♥ to ensure it is safe to start cardiac rehabilitation after a heart attack, heart surgery, angioplasty, or stent placement

♥ to see if you will need a heart transplant if you have had heart failure

♥ to assess your response to therapy if you have pulmonary hypertension

An exercise stress test is not the test for everyone. Anyone with severe aortic stenosis, unstable angina, an ECG abnormality known as a left bundle branch block, or anyone who cannot exercise should not undergo an exercise stress test.

Nearly two-thirds of heart attack deaths in women occur among those who have no history of chest pain.

Results: Test interpretation depends on why the test was ordered. In general, if your doctor is looking for reduced blood flow to your heart, all the factors monitored may reveal it: the exercise duration, ECG, blood pressure response, heart rate response, and heart rate recovery, in addition to the symptoms you may experience during the test. If your stress test is abnormal, you may be advised to undergo another stress test with imaging, or you may require an *angiogram* (*cardiac catheterization*) to assess for coronary artery blockages.

No test, of course, is perfect. It is possible that some stress test results, such as ECG changes, may be falsely positive, meaning that what appears to suggest reduced blood flow to the heart is actually not that. But data can help doctors determine how perfect (and imperfect) a test is and help put the results into the context of the pre-test suspicion. For instance, if your symptoms suggest heart disease, your doctor will be more likely to believe a positive result. Imaging is used to make the test more accurate, as discussed in the next section.

Risks: As its name implies, this test stresses the heart. And so there is a risk of causing a heart attack. There is also a risk of inducing angina or reproducing the symptoms that suggested the test was needed, which can be difficult to control in some cases and can cause unstable angina. An exercise stress test can also induce a cardiac arrhythmia.

Because of these risks, a physician must supervise your stress test to watch for anything concerning and stop the test when appropriate. He or she will monitor you not only throughout the test but also during the test recovery period.

Echocardiogram Stress Test

Method: An *echocardiogram* (echo) *stress test* can be done using an exercise stress test or a *pharmacologic stress test* (where you don't exercise but are given an injection of the drug dobutamine to increase the heart rate and mimic what occurs with exercise). No matter which method is used, an ultrasound probe is placed on the chest to take images of the heart at both rest and stress, in order to compare the wall motion of the ventricle of the heart. Images may also be taken at any point during stress, as well as during the recovery phase. The echocardiogram images with stress are used to assess heart valve function. You should not drink caffeine before this test, and you may be asked to not take certain medications prior to testing.

Purpose: The following are possible reasons for undergoing an echocardiogram stress testing:
- ♥ to check for coronary heart disease, usually because of symptoms of chest pressure, chest pain, shortness of breath with exertion, or any symptoms that make your doctor concerned about reduced blood flow to the heart muscle — particularly if an ECG abnormality makes the ECG with stress testing unreliable on its own and imaging is required to accurately assess for ischemia
- ♥ to check for coronary artery disease based on an abnormality on an ECG, where an ECG abnormality makes the ECG with stress testing unreliable on its own and imaging is required to accurately assess for ischemia
- ♥ to test the effectiveness of any procedure (e.g., coronary artery bypass surgery or placement of a coronary artery stent or angioplasty) that has been done to improve blood flow to the heart

♥ to look for heart valve abnormalities with stress to determine the possible need for surgery

Pharmacologic stress testing is required for women who cannot exercise but need their coronary arteries assessed for any of the reasons we've outlined here.

Results: A physician will review your response to stress on the ECG, as well as review your echo images. A normal response is a uniform increase in contraction of all walls of the left ventricle with stress. An area that does not contract well with stress suggests reduced blood flow in that particular coronary artery area. In addition, blood flow over a narrowed (*stenosed*) or leaky (*regurgitant*) heart valve can be assessed to measure its severity with stress, which may be found to be more significant than what the reported symptoms suggest.

Risks: The same risk exists in an echocardiogram stress test as for exercise stress testing (see above) if exercise is used to stress the heart. With pharmacologic stress, additional risks may exist because of the drug used to induce stress, which may also induce ischemia.

Nuclear Stress Test

Method: *Nuclear stress testing*, also known as *SPECT* (single photon emission computed tomography) imaging, can be done using an exercise stress test or a pharmacologic stress test. A radioactive isotope is injected through a vein to assess the blood flow to the heart under stress. The findings are then compared to a similar image of the heart at rest. Typically, the two isotopes that are injected are *thallium* for the resting images and *technetium* for the stress images, but more recently we are using technetium alone for both images (rest and stress) in order to reduce the amount of radiation. A *gamma camera*, which detects gamma rays from the body after it has been given a radioactive drug, takes pictures after each image to show the blood flow to the heart muscle. If there is a coronary artery with significant blockage, this will often show up as an area of the heart with poor blood flow when the heart is stressed compared to at rest.

A pharmacologic nuclear stress test usually involves injecting drugs that cause increased blood flow by dilating or relaxing (*vasodilation*) the coronary arteries. The drugs commonly used are adenosine (Adenoscan) or regadenoson (Lexiscan). An older drug and one rarely used today is dipyridamole. When adenosine or regadenoson cannot be used, dobutamine may be used to mimic stress by raising the heart rate. When undergoing a stress test, it is important to tell the doctor administering the test if you have asthma or a history of heart block, so he or she can choose the right drug for you. Don't drink caffeine before any stress test, as it will make certain drugs ineffective. Talk to your doctor if you have any concerns about the effects of the drugs used in the testing.

Purpose: Your doctor might order nuclear stress testing for the following reasons:
- ♥ to check for coronary heart disease, usually because of symptoms of chest pressure, chest pain, shortness of breath with exertion, or any symptoms that make your doctor concerned about reduced blood flow to the heart muscle — particularly if an ECG abnormality makes the ECG with stress testing unreliable on its own and imaging is required to accurately assess for ischemia
- ♥ to check for coronary artery disease — need for the test may be based on an abnormality discovered on an ECG if the abnormality makes the ECG with stress testing unreliable on its own and imaging is required to accurately assess for ischemia
- ♥ to test the effectiveness of any procedure (coronary artery bypass surgery or placement of a coronary artery stent or angioplasty) that has been done to improve blood flow to the heart
- ♥ presence of a left bundle branch block on the ECG at baseline — then pharmacologic (adenosine) nuclear stress test is the test of choice

Results: A nuclear stress test is also known as a *perfusion stress test*. This means the test can assess the blood flow (*perfusion*) to the heart with stress compared to rest. Normal results are when the blood flow increases to the heart uniformly (to all walls of the left ventricle equally).

Risks: The same risks exist as for exercise stress testing (see the previous test) if exercise is used to stress the heart. With pharmacologic stress, additional risks exist because of the drugs used to induce stress.

There is some radiation exposure with this test, but there is less radiation if technetium is used at rest and stress.

Positron Emission Tomography

Method: *Positron emission tomography,* or a *PET scan,* is a type of nuclear stress test that creates a 3-D image of the heart to assess its function when it is under stress. A radioactive sugar is injected intravenously as a tracer; the organs take about an hour to take in the sugar so that it appears in the scan. You'll be advised not to smoke, eat, or drink anything containing caffeine for four to six hours before the test, so that nothing interferes with how the radioactive tracer is distributed in the body. PET stress testing provides more detailed images than standard nuclear stress testing, but its high cost generally outweighs its usefulness, unless standard nuclear imaging fails to properly assess for ischemia. PET imaging is particularly useful in determining if the heart muscle is alive after a heart attack, where there is chronic blockage in coronary arteries, or where there has been damage or scarring to the heart. It may also be particularly useful in women with large breasts or in those who are obese to assess the heart more accurately than any other type of stress testing.

Purpose: Used for the same purposes as SPECT, which we discussed in the previous section.

Results: The physician will interpret the result in the same manner as a SPECT.

Risks: Similar to nuclear stress testing, as described above. There is some radiation exposure with this test. If you are pregnant, please inform the supervising physician of this fact.

Multi-Gated Acquisition Scan

Method: A *multi-gated acquisition scan,* also known as a *MUGA scan* or a *gated blood pool examination,* involves an intravenous injection of a radioactive isotope (technetium), which is either mixed with the person's blood ahead of time or is preceded by an injection of tin before being injected. A gamma camera takes a series of images of the heart during one complete cardiac cycle (one heartbeat). These images show the blood pooling in the heart chambers over the cardiac cycle, and the quantity of blood the heart is able to squeeze out over one cardiac cycle (the heart's *ejection fraction*) is mathematically calculated.

Purpose: MUGA scans are used to evaluate the function of the right and left ventricles. These can be compared to images done previously, to assess for changes over time. These scans are often used on women with breast cancer before they undergo chemotherapy as it may be toxic to the heart. Two drugs that are used to treat breast cancer and which can affect the heart are doxorubicin (Adriamycin) and trastuzumab (Herceptin). And so, a MUGA scan is routinely done before using these drugs and then again during treatment, or if symptoms appear at any time after chemotherapy, to detect the possibility of heart failure.

Results: The results of a MUGA scan are accurate, reproducible, and highly reliable. Normal results are when all the heart walls are moving normally and the ejection fraction is approximately 60% (or in the range of 50 to 80%), since the normal heart squeezes forward about 60% of the blood it receives in total. An abnormal result is when it appears that some areas of the heart are either not contracting at all or contracting less than they should (*abnormal wall motion*) or if the heart's ejection fraction is less than 50%.

Risks: With a MUGA scan there is a risk of radiation exposure from the technetium. If you are pregnant, please inform the supervising physician of this fact.

Magnetic Resonance Imaging

Method: *Magnetic Resonance Imaging* (*MRI*) uses a magnetic field and radio frequency pulses to produce detailed images of the heart and its surrounding structures. MRI allows physicians to evaluate the various parts of the heart and their functions, including the heart muscle, the surrounding pericardium, the heart valves, the coronary arteries, and the great vessels coming off the heart. Sometimes an intravenous injection of a contrast medium (*gadolinium*) is used for an MRI. This screening method produces images of the heart and its function over time, so you would be asked to lie flat inside a large cylinder-shaped scanner, where a circular magnet surrounds you, and you would need to keep as still as possible for about 30 minutes. Some people cannot undergo this test, such as those with certain metal implants: a pacemaker, defibrillator, cochlear ear implant, mechanical heart valve, some types of clips used to treat brain aneurysms, and bullets or shrapnel, depending on their location in the body. Also, orthopedic implants do affect MRI scanning. Make sure the radiologist or technician doing the test is aware of any metal you may have in your body (but, typically, they'll ask you ahead of time).

Purpose: An MRI scan is often ordered if other testing methods, such as an echocardiogram, X-ray, or CT scan, have been unable to answer a specific question regarding the heart. MRI can be done to more accurately assess heart function, check for congenital abnormalities, measure ventricular wall thickness, and look at coronary blood flow. In addition, it is often used to assess blood flow to the heart and the viability of the heart muscle after a heart attack to determine if there is damaged and permanent scarring or if there is some viable functioning heart muscle. The MRI will help the cardiologist to determine if the heart muscle could benefit from revascularization with a coronary artery stent or cardiac bypass surgery, or if the heart is damaged beyond such repair.

Results: The resulting images will be read by a cardiologist, radiologist, or both, looking to answer the indication for this test — that is, what caused the test to be ordered — in addition to reviewing any other information they see on the images.

Risks: There is no radiation exposure with MRI. If you are anxious or claustrophobic, it may be hard for you to be in the cylindrical tube, and it might help to ask for a sedative ahead of time. There is a rare, but possible, risk of damage to the kidneys if gadolinium is injected, but this seems to be most common in persons with very poor kidney function. MRI appears to be safe to use in pregnancy, but be sure to tell your doctor if you are pregnant before undergoing the test. A pregnant woman should have an MRI only if the benefits outweigh the slight but possible risks this powerful magnetic field poses to the fetus.

MRI with Stress Testing
Method: A stress test with MRI uses the same MRI technology as described in the previous section but involves an active stress test to assess for heart muscle blood flow during stress compared to a resting state.

Stress MRI is much more expensive that a regular stress test with any other type of imaging, so it is only used for certain indications. Because you need to be very still during an MRI, an injection of adenosine (Adenoscan) will usually be given to induce stress, increasing blood flow by dilating or relaxing (*vasodilating*) the coronary arteries once you're inside the scanner. Resting images are obtained first and then stress images are captured. More recently, physicians and researchers at Ohio State University have developed a protocol to perform an exercise stress test and then, using MRI, capture images quickly after that exercise.[1] Like a standard exercise stress test, an ECG is monitored throughout exercise, but at the end of exercise, you are quickly moved to an MRI scanner in the same room. This method is likely to become more popular because it does not require the use of drugs and it allows physicians to collect the important diagnostic and prognostic information that comes from exercise stress testing. The images from a cardiac MRI stress test appear to be better than those from other imaging methods — without any radiation exposure. An MRI stress test takes about 35 minutes. Don't eat or drink caffeine before the test.

Purpose: The following are indications for MRI stress testing:

♥ To check for coronary heart disease where the usual methods of stress testing show nothing, but symptoms suggest reduced blood flow to the heart muscle.

♥ To check for coronary artery disease for women who require stress testing with imaging.

♥ To test the effectiveness of any procedure (coronary artery bypass surgery or placement of a coronary artery stent or angioplasty) that has been done to improve blood flow to the heart.

♥ When *Cardiac Syndrome X*, a condition that most frequently occurs in women, is present. Cardiac Syndrome X is defined as the presence of chest pain and evidence of ischemia, but no evidence of obstructive coronary artery disease by an angiogram. Often an initial stress test using standard methods (exercise ECG, exercise or pharmacologic stress test with echo or nuclear imaging) reveals abnormal results and suggests ischemia, yet an angiogram to look for coronary artery blockages is normal. It is believed that Cardiac Syndrome X may be due to small vessel disease (*microvascular ischemia*) that cannot be seen on an angiogram (a test we discuss near the end of this chapter), or possibly due to an abnormal response of the blood vessels to stress (*endothelial dysfunction*). This may affect the muscle in the innermost area of the heart (*endocardium*) and may be best detected by an MRI stress test.

> The plaque in men's arteries distributes itself in clumps, whereas in many cases the plaque in women's arteries seems to distribute itself more evenly throughout artery walls. This results in women's angiographic studies being misinterpreted as normal.

Results: Blood flow to the heart muscle (*myocardium*) is assessed at rest and during stress and the results are compared. Decreased blood flow to an area of the heart is consistent with *ischemia* (reduced blood flow to the heart). The pattern of the reduced blood flow may suggest that there is a narrowed coronary artery or a more diffuse process, such as endothelial dysfunction or microvascular ischemia.

Risks: The same risks exist as for exercise stress testing (see pages 58 to 60) if exercise is used to stress the heart. With pharmacologic stress, there are additional risks because of the drug used to induce stress. We described the risk related to MRI earlier in this chapter.

Ankle-Brachial Index (ABI) Test

Method: The *ankle-brachial index* (ABI) test can be easily done in a clinic or hospital if your medical history or an exam suggests *peripheral arterial disease* (PAD, the clogging of arteries in the body), especially in the legs. The ABI compares blood pressure between lower extremities (legs) and upper extremities (arms). Normally, blood pressure is higher in the legs than the arms, so when this is not the case, it suggests *peripheral vascular disease* (PVD). ABI values are measured by applying an inflatable cuff to the calf and then to the upper arm. The systolic blood pressure reading of the calf is divided by that of the arm. Sometimes an ultrasound device (*Doppler probe*) is used to detect the systolic blood pressure for increased accuracy.

Purpose: The test will be done if you have symptoms of *claudication* (leg pain while you walk or even when you're at rest) or signs suggesting reduced blood flow to one or both legs. The ABI should be assessed in anyone with preexisting cardiovascular disease of any type (coronary, cerebral, or kidney arterial disease). The test should also be performed as a screening in those over the age of 70, or in those between the ages of 50 and 69 who smoke or are diabetic, even if they have no symptoms of PAD.

Results: A normal ABI value is one that is higher than 1. An ABI value less than 0.9 is considered abnormal and indicates reduced systolic blood pressure to the legs, compared with the arms, suggesting peripheral arterial disease (see the table below). This test can be less accurate in some people with diabetes or kidney disease and in elderly persons, and the test results may need to be confirmed with an MRI or CT scan. The following table shows a range of ABI values and what they mean.

Ankle-Brachial Index

Result	ABI value
Normal	>0.90
Mild PAD	>0.80 to <0.90
Moderate PAD	0.40 to 0.80
Severe PAD	<0.40

Risks: None.

Carotid Ultrasound

Method: A *carotid ultrasound* uses sound waves to make images of the *carotid arteries*, the two major arteries that carry blood from the heart to the brain. These arteries, the right and the left, provide blood to their respective sides of the brain. Part of the ultrasound examination will be to assess blood flow through the arteries using a Doppler probe.

Purpose: This test may be done if you have had a stroke or a *transient ischemic attack* (TIA, which is considered a small stroke without any permanent damage). It may be done when a *carotid bruit* (an abnormal noise heard over the artery when listened to with a stethoscope) is detected in either or both carotid arteries. Often, a carotid ultrasound is done after a carotid stent is placed to open a narrowed carotid artery to assess blood flow in the artery and the position of the stent. It can also be performed on a person who is at very high risk for cerebrovascular disease.

Results: A carotid ultrasound will show if there is plaque in either carotid artery that has caused narrowing (*stenosis*) and is causing reduced blood flow to the brain. Plaque is evidence of *carotid artery disease* (also known as *cerebrovascular disease*). Excessive plaque in the carotid arteries can result in a stroke.

Risks: None.

> Of the 795,000 strokes that occur each year in the United States, about 185,000 are recurrent strokes.

Carotid Intima-Medial Thickness

Method: Also known as a *carotid IMT*, this test is performed using an ultrasound as described in the previous section, but this ultrasound is specifically measuring the thickness of the carotid artery wall. The thickening of the carotid walls is strongly associated with an increased risk of atherosclerosis. This test can be done as part of the carotid ultrasound.

Purpose: The use of this test to assess risk of cardiovascular disease is strongly supported by the American Heart Association and the U.S.-based National Cholesterol Education Program, Third Adult Treatment Panel.[2]

Results: A way to think about the result of a carotid IMT is that it is the closest "window" to the heart, providing a simple view of the risk to the coronary arteries that carry blood to your heart. The baseline assessment of carotid IMT has important prognostic information about your future risk of coronary artery disease, as does the change in your carotid IMT over time. Typical baseline measurements of carotid IMT range between 0.6 and 1.0 millimeters (mm) and a typical progression rate of carotid IMT over time is about 0.01 mm per year. When carotid IMT has increased 0.1 mm or more a year, there is a significant increased risk of heart problems. The carotid IMT results appear to improve the accuracy of predicting the risk when considered in addition to traditional cardiac risk factors.

Risks: None.

Computed Tomography (CT) Heart Scan

Method: A *computed tomography* (*CT*) scan is a type of X-ray that repeatedly takes thin, cross-sectional images of your heart, or *tomograms*. These "slices" are then reconstructed on a computer to produce a detailed image of the heart. Usually you will be injected with a contrast dye during the scan so that the coronary arteries of the heart can be better assessed. The CT scanner is a large X-ray machine with a short tube that acquires the images quickly (in up to 10 seconds). Some CT scanners — the electron beam CT (EBCT) and 64-slice CT scanner, for example — are even faster than the older type of scanner. The effect of the heart's motion is minimized because they are so quick.

Purpose: CT heart scans are often used to screen for heart disease and assess the amount of calcium in the coronary arteries. They are often promoted as screening for heart disease, but generally other tests are needed as a result of CT findings, because the significance or implications of the findings aren't always clear and the CT test is not covered by most insurance plans. Although CT heart scans can be done for reasons other than looking at coronary calcium, they are usually done to assess the aorta for an aortic dissection (if symptoms are present) or if there has been trauma to the chest area. Similarly, a CT scan may be done to assess for an aortic aneurysm. A CT scan may be done to create imagery of the pulmonary veins before an *atrial fibrillation ablation* procedure. (*Atrial fibrillation* is the most common type of heart arrhythmia and puts one at risk of stroke; *ablation* is the procedure whereby the source of the fibrillation is destroyed, most commonly by "burning" it with radiofrequency energy to prevent the arrhythmia from recurring.) A CT scan can also be used to assess the pericardium of the heart and to diagnose a *pulmonary embolism* (blockage of a lung artery with a blood clot that has traveled through the right side of the heart).

Results: As a screening tool, a CT scan cannot predict immediate risks to the heart, even if it indicates that coronary calcium is present. Doing so requires additional testing (often a stress test and possibly an angiogram) to determine if any narrowing in an artery is significantly reducing the blood flow to the heart. Nonetheless, coronary artery calcium is a significant predictor of future cardiac events. *Calcification* in the coronary arteries is calcified plaque that has been present for some time. And so the risk of this calcified plaque rupturing and causing a heart attack is less likely than a fresh, soft plaque that is not detected by this method. But a CT scan will show excessive blockage in a coronary artery, which means that the risk of a heart attack is higher compared to someone with no coronary artery calcium. And, of course, the more calcium that is present, the greater the risk for heart disease, over time.

Softer, non-calcified plaque appears be more concerning in terms of a possible imminent heart attack, but the technology to assess the presence of soft plaque in the arteries is still being developed and is not yet widely available. The technology is promising and will likely become more widely available soon, although whether it should be used in everyone as a screening tool remains to be seen. And that is a question we need answered before women get needless radiation and excess testing (and quite possibly more radiation). Routine use of heart scans on women who don't have any symptoms of heart disease is not recommended by the American Heart Association or the American College of Cardiology, and a CT scan in particular is not a test that needs to be done repeatedly to assess risk over time.

Risks: There is radiation exposure during this test. A CT scan will focus on your left breast, as this is the area over your heart, and so radiation is concentrated there. If contrast dye is given with the CT scan, there may be risks related to the dye that your physician will explain prior to the procedure.

Tilt Table Test
Method: You'll be asked to stop taking any medications prior to the test and to fast for at least six hours. You'll be asked to lie down and you'll be strapped to a flat board. An intravenous line will be placed in your arm, in case you need to be given medication quickly. Then you'll be turned upright, as if standing. An ECG will be recorded, as will blood pressure, pulse, blood oxygen levels, and any symptoms you experience with this change in position. If you do not pass out with this, you might be given a drug (isoproterenol or glycerine trinitrate)

to increase the chance of passing out and the tilt table part of the test will be repeated.

Purpose: This test is used when a person has had an episode where she has passed out (*syncope*) or experienced lightheadedness, dizziness, or the sensation of almost passing out (*presyncope*) and the cause is not clear — the test is done to try to induce the symptoms.

Results: Normally, a person's blood pressure will not dramatically change when moving from a lying down to a completely upright position (after all, we jump out of bed many times and we don't all pass out!). The body quickly compensates for changes in position by increasing the heart rate and constricting blood vessels to increase blood return to the heart. A tilt table test has a positive result if the patient experiences symptoms associated with a drop in blood pressure or a cardiac arrhythmia, or passes out. In general, a positive tilt test is consistent with a diagnosis of *vasovagal syncope* (also known as *postural hypotension* or *neurocardiogenic syncope*). This occurs when the autonomic nervous system is not functioning normally and is not responding to a particular trigger quickly enough. Triggers can be any number of things, including standing up quickly, prolonged standing, stress, pain, nervousness, arousal, dehydration, and urinating or having a bowel movement.

Risks: One risk is that a person can pass out during the test and, rarely, the heart can stop or a seizure can even occur. However, the test is closely monitored and if any adverse event occurs, you'll be treated quickly. Often laying the person back down can resolve any issues, but occasionally fluid and medication will be needed to reverse an adverse event.

Ambulatory Blood Pressure Monitor

Method: An *ambulatory blood pressure monitor* is a portable monitor that you wear for about 24 hours. It assesses your blood pressure at equal intervals throughout the day. The monitor consists of an arm cuff and a small pack (about the size of a pager) worn on your belt. As you wear the monitor, go about your daily routine and keep a diary to record any symptoms.

Purpose: An ambulatory blood pressure cuff is used in the following situations:

♥ if it is unclear whether your blood pressure is truly elevated or elevated only in your doctor's office (also known as *white coat hypertension* — discussed in Chapter 2)

♥ if you have prehypertension and it is unclear if your blood pressure is higher at points in your day other than during your doctor's visit

♥ if your blood pressure is poorly controlled, despite the fact that you're taking medication to control it

♥ if you are pregnant and have hypertension

♥ if you have fainting spells (*syncope*)

Results: Each blood pressure reading over the 24-hour period is documented and reported to help you and your doctor assess whether you need treatment or assistance to improve your blood pressure.

Risks: None.

Holter Monitor

Method: A *Holter monitor* is basically an ambulatory electrocardiogram (ECG) that assesses the heart's rate and rhythm for a certain period, often 24 or 48 hours. Electrodes are placed on the chest and a recording device (about the size of a pager) is also strapped to the chest (it can be worn under loose clothing). You'll be instructed to do your normal daily activities, particularly those that may trigger your symptoms. You'll also be asked to keep a diary and record any symptoms while wearing the Holter monitor.

Purpose: This is a useful tool to diagnose symptoms that occur almost daily. A Holter monitor is used for the following reasons:

♥ when a person is experiencing *palpitations* (awareness of heartbeat) or a "fluttering in the chest" sensation, particularly when these palpitations are irregular, fast, or both

♥ when a person has symptoms of passing out or almost passing out (*syncope* or *presyncope*), lightheadedness, or dizziness

♥ when a slow heart rate needs to be assessed

♥ when a person is starting certain heart medications

♥ after a heart attack — if there is concern that an arrhythmia may be present

♥ if a person has had cardiac surgery and if atrial fibrillation occurred — the monitor will assess if atrial fibrillation is still present or coming and going

Results: A normal result is when no abnormalities are recorded during the period the monitor is worn, aside from the normal variations in heart rate that occur during daily activities. But this doesn't necessarily mean that everything is normal, as the problem may not occur during the period the Holter is worn. If you did not experience any of your symptoms while wearing the monitor, let your doctor know. An abnormal result is when an irregular heart rate or rhythm is captured on the monitor, due to an arrhythmia. There are many types of abnormal heart rhythms, some too fast, some too slow, some with risks of blood clots, and some that can be quite dangerous if not treated. Once the monitor captures abnormal heart rhythms, your doctor will know which is the cause of your symptoms and be better able to direct further testing or treatment.

Risks: None.

Event Monitor
Method: An *event monitor* is an ambulatory electrocardiogram (ECG) that is typically worn for 30 days to record the heart rate and rhythm "on demand." Some event monitors can detect changes from normal and will record automatically. Others require the person wearing the monitor to trigger the recording. (The first type is preferred, especially for brief arrhythmias.) And some event monitors can even transfer recorded information via telephone so that it can be interpreted quickly. Electrodes are placed on the chest and a recording device (about the size of a deck of cards) is strapped to the chest (this can be worn under loose clothing). You'll be instructed to do your normal activities, particularly activities that may trigger your symptoms. You'll also be asked to keep a diary and record any symptoms.

Purpose: An event monitor is a useful tool to diagnose symptoms that occur unpredictably, irregularly, and infrequently (weekly or even less often). It is used for the following reasons:

♥ if a person is experiencing the same symptoms as a Holter monitor is used for (see the previous section), but the symptoms occur sporadically, unpredictably, and infrequently
♥ when a Holter monitor has failed to record any abnormality but the symptoms persist

Results: A cardiologist will interpret the heart rhythms tracing that the monitor produces. If symptoms occur and the heart rhythm is normal, that is considered a normal event and you'll know that the symptoms are not due to an arrhythmia. Abnormal results range from simple skipped heartbeats that are variants of normal to dangerous arrhythmias that can be life-threatening.

Risks: None.

Invasive Tests

Invasive tests are those where instruments are inserted into the body. Usually they are ordered after noninvasive tests have abnormal results.

Angiogram (Cardiac Catheterizations)

Method: An *angiogram*, also known as a *cardiac catheterization* or a "cath" for short, is a common procedure. It is an invasive test where a cardiologist can have a direct look at the heart arteries. To access the coronary arteries, a small tube is inserted in a *femoral artery* (near the crease of your groin, on either side, where your leg appears to meet your hip), but sometimes the artery in your arm can be used rather than the femoral artery. A thin wire guides a long tube (a *catheter*) through a shorter tube up from the access artery, to the aorta, and toward the heart. The wire is removed and the catheter is positioned so that the tip is resting in a coronary artery. Contrast dye is injected to show the artery and the image is captured on film, using an X-ray. You will need to fast for 12 hours before the procedure and you'll also be advised in advance which medications you must take and which you cannot. Diabetics on a particular medication or those with some kidney damage may be required by the doctor to take medication before the procedure to protect the kidneys. You will be awake during the test, but you may get a mild sedative if you are nervous.

Once a catheter is in place, depending on the findings, an *angioplasty* may be done, which is where a balloon is inserted into the blockage in the heart artery and temporarily inflated to open the blocked artery. This is often followed by a *stent* placement — a metal, coil-like spring that is expanded in the heart artery to keep a blocked artery open.

Purpose: An angiogram may be done for the following reasons:
- ♥ to directly assess the degree of blockage in a coronary artery
- ♥ to confirm that a heart attack has occurred and to assess the coronary artery involved and the extent of damage to the heart muscle
- ♥ to determine the course of treatment after a heart attack or for those with unstable angina
- ♥ to determine the degree of coronary artery disease after an abnormal cardiac stress test
- ♥ to assess heart valve function
- ♥ to assess heart muscle function
- ♥ to determine blood pressure in the heart and oxygen levels of the blood in the heart chambers

Results: The images captured by an angiogram allow the doctor to assess blockages in the coronary arteries. Contrast dye is injected to show the blood flow in the coronary artery and the artery segments are compared to areas preceding and following it. If it is unclear if there is a significant blockage, an *intravascular ultrasound* (IVUS) may be inserted to assess the artery in more detail. If there is no blockage, the test result is considered normal. An abnormal result means there is a blockage in the heart artery. In general, only a significant blockage of 70% or more will require any intervention beyond medical treatment.

Risks: Minor risks are related to mild bruising or bleeding at the access site on your arm or leg. Major complications are rare. Nonetheless, there is a less than 1% risk of an angiogram inducing heart attack, stroke, peripheral artery clot, embolism, major bleeding, or death. The risk increases to 1% if a stent or angioplasty is done during the angiogram. Some people are allergic to the contrast dye, and people who have had a past allergic reaction to a contrast agent, iodine, or shellfish will be treated in advance to prevent such a reaction. There is radiation exposure from any angiogram, and the amount of radiation will vary depending on the length of the procedure, the number of X-rays required, and if an intervention (angioplasty/stent) was performed.

Women with heart attacks or unstable or stable angina are less likely to be referred for angiography than are men with the same diagnoses. It is debatable whether this reflects underuse of angiography in women or overuse in men.

Electrophysiology Study with or without Cardiac Ablation

Method: An *electrophysiology study* (*EP study*) is a test of the heart's electrical system. Usually two to three catheters are inserted into either the groin or neck blood vessels to get access to the heart. The catheters are placed in the heart with the guidance of an X-ray, like that used in an angiogram. The catheters are insulated wires with metal electrodes. Once the catheters are positioned, they record the electrical signals in the heart. They can also be used to control the heart rate and where the heartbeat starts, thereby allowing the doctor to study the electrical system and see whether it responds normally or abnormally. You will be asked to fast for about 12 hours before the test and you will also be instructed on which medications you should or should not take. Usually medications that might suppress a heart rhythm abnormality will be stopped in advance of the test.

Purpose: An EP study is used to study both slow heart rhythms (*bradyarrhythmias*) and fast heart rhythms (*tachyarrhythmias*). The finding of certain arrhythmias will make it clear if a pacemaker is needed, which can be placed at the time of the EP study. Other arrhythmias can be treated with an ablation procedure during the EP study if the origin of the problem has been identified. In this procedure the source of the arrhythmia is destroyed, for example, by burning it with radiofrequency energy; this is often done at the time of the study to minimize the need for further procedures and limit the patient's radiation exposure. Occasionally, a dangerous arrhythmia — that can cause sudden cardiac death — can be identified and may require insertion of a defibrillator, which will be done at the time of the study.

Results: A cardiologist who specializes in heart rhythm problems (an *electrophysiologist*) will perform the tests and interpret the results at the time of testing.

Risks: The potential risks of having an EP study are similar to those of having a cardiac catheterization (see earlier in this chapter). Although usually only minor bleeding and bruising occur at the site of access, the major risks are more serious bleeding, perforation of the heart wall resulting in something called *cardiac tamponade* (compression of the heart), or cardiac arrest. Major risks are estimated to be 1 in 1000, similar to that of a cardiac catheterization. Because X-ray images are taken, there is radiation exposure with any EP study. How much radiation you are exposed to depends on the length of the study.

The Heart of the Matter

The most common way people give up their power is by thinking they don't have any.

— Alice Walker

Many tests can be done to screen for heart disease; here we have focused on the most common tests that are used routinely. Some tests determine your immediate risk, but others also provide important information for the future. Always make sure you know why a test is being performed. You should know both the benefits of getting the test and the risks involved. Be sure to ask your doctor any questions you may have before the test is done, and once the test results are available, discuss with your doctor what the results mean. (It is our job as physicians to translate that risk to you in a meaningful way, and you have a right to know and understand test results.) Then discuss what next steps you will take.

Do not be scared of tests. If having a certain test will help get to the bottom of your symptoms or better assess your risk of heart problems, it is worthwhile. But don't interpret the test result as a "pass" or "fail." Even if you get a diagnosis of heart disease, a heart arrhythmia, or anything else, the fact is that having the information empowers you to change your outcome for the better. Ignorance is only bliss until you realize you have no time to make changes that can prolong your life.

Chapter 5

Heart Medications

Medicine is not only a science; it is also an art. It does not consist of compounding pills and plasters; it deals with the very processes of life, which must be understood before they may be guided.
— Philippus A. Paracelsus

Modern medicine has come a long way over the past few decades. We have gained tremendous understanding about the causes and risk factors for chronic diseases such as heart disease, as well as how to treat and prevent them.

It is true that heart disease is largely preventable. In the coming chapters we discuss the role of nutrition, exercise, stress management, and other key factors for prevention. But for some women, lifestyle modifications alone are not enough. For those who have developed a form of heart disease or are at high risk because of genetics, medications may be necessary to manage symptoms and prevent potentially fatal consequences like heart attack or stroke.

No one likes to leave the doctor's office with a prescription — unless it is a prescription for a vacation! The idea of taking medication for life can be a hard pill to swallow. It can be challenging to manage the costs and side effects, and remembering to take medication every day is not easy. We hear these concerns constantly from our patients. Nevertheless, if you have suffered a heart attack or stroke, are considered at high risk for heart disease, or have a serious heart condition, you will likely be prescribed medication to manage your condition, and you will need to take most of these medications for the rest of your life. Taking these medications *as prescribed* can literally mean the difference between life and death.

It is important to be aware that finding the right drug(s) to manage your particular condition may require some fine-tuning. Medicine is both an art and a science. And because everyone reacts differently to medication, the type of drug you are prescribed and the dosage may require adjusting in order for your therapy to be optimized.

Medicine is a science of uncertainty and an art of probability.
—William Osler

Types of Heart Drugs

In this section you'll find key information about the various classes of heart medications — the good (benefits), the bad (side effects), the ugly (serious risks), and the noteworthy (special precautions, including potential interactions with foods and supplements). Since most drugs have more than one name, we have indicated the chemical name of the drug, followed by the brand name in parentheses. We've listed the most commonly prescribed medications in each category.

There are many potential interactions between drugs, ranging from minor to severe, and it is not possible to list all the interactions here. Nor have we listed all possible side effects. We highlighted those that are most common and concerning. It is always best to check with your pharmacist when you are prescribed a new medication, especially if you get prescriptions filled at more than one pharmacy and/or are seeing more than one doctor.

ACE (Angiotensin-Converting Enzyme) Inhibitors

♥ benazepril (Lotensin)
♥ captopril (Capoten)
♥ enalapril (Vasotec)
♥ fosinopril (Monopril)
♥ lisinopril (Prinivil, Zestril)
♥ quinapril (Accupril)
♥ ramipril (Altace)
♥ trandolapril (Mavik)

The Good

ACE inhibitors dilate the blood vessels to increase the amount of blood the heart pumps and to lower blood pressure. ACE inhibitors also increase blood flow, which helps to decrease the workload on the heart. Another important effect of ACE inhibitors is that they prevent dangerous remodelling of the heart that can occur after a heart attack or in heart failure.

These drugs are often prescribed to treat high blood pressure and heart failure and to prevent heart attack and stroke for those at high risk. They are also given to people after a heart attack to prevent damage to the heart and improve survival rate, and they may be given to diabetics to help slow or prevent kidney damage.

The Bad

The most common side effect of ACE inhibitors is a persistent dry cough, but this class of medication can also cause nausea, headache, diarrhea, constipation, dizziness or lightheadedness, a salty/metallic taste in the mouth, or a temporary loss of taste.

The Ugly

Angioedema is a rare but serious side effect of ACE inhibitors. This condition causes swelling of the skin and tissues of the face, lips, mouth, throat, and extremities. Angioedema can be life-threatening if it involves the larynx. If you are taking an ACE inhibitor and experience any swelling, contact your doctor immediately or go to the closest hospital.

The Noteworthy

♥ Avoid using salt substitutes when taking an ACE inhibitor. Salt substitutes contain potassium, and ACE inhibitors cause the body to retain potassium. High potassium levels (*hyperkalemia*) can be harmful to your heart and kidneys.

♥ Over-the-counter non-steroidal anti-inflammatory medications (such as Motrin or Advil) and aspirin may cause the body to retain salt and water and decrease the efficacy of an ACE inhibitor. Check with your doctor or pharmacist before taking any anti-inflammatory medications or other over-the-counter medications or supplements.

♥ ACE inhibitors can deplete zinc levels in the body. This can potentially cause slow wound-healing, impair smell and taste, and lower immunity.

♥ While taking an ACE inhibitor, have your blood pressure and kidney function checked regularly, as recommended by your doctor.
♥ Women should NOT be on an ACE inhibitor if they plan to get pregnant or are pregnant.

Aldosterone Inhibitors
♥ eplerenone (Inspra)
♥ spironolactone (Aldactone)

The Good
Also known as potassium-sparing diuretics, these drugs block *aldosterone*, a natural substance in the body that causes salt and fluid buildup and stiffening of the heart muscle. By lowering the amount of salt and water your body retains they can help lower blood pressure. Both eplerenone and spironolactone are prescribed for people with high blood pressure and chronic heart failure to improve outcomes and to prevent symptoms from becoming worse. This class of drug may also be prescribed for those who develop left ventricular dysfunction following a heart attack, as it may prevent heart muscle damage from worsening.

The Bad
The most common side effects of aldosterone inhibitors may include headache, dizziness, upset stomach, fatigue, breast enlargement or tenderness, and abnormal vaginal bleeding.

The Ugly
Serious side effects of these drugs may include confusion, irregular heartbeat, numbness, tingling or weakness in the hands or feet, chest pain, or cold, gray skin. Contact your doctor immediately if you experience any of these symptoms.

The Noteworthy
♥ Increased urination while taking these drugs is normal and may last for up to six hours after a dose.
♥ Avoid potassium supplements, salt substitutes containing potassium, and eating large amounts of potassium-rich foods such as bananas and orange juice because these drugs can raise your body's potassium levels, which can cause irregular heart rhythm and affect the function of the heart.

♥ Potassium levels should be closely monitored when aldosterone inhibtors are taken in conjunction with ACE Inhibitors or ARBs, since all can raise potassium levels.

♥ Supplements that may interact with these drugs include St. John's wort, arginine, white willow, and zinc.

Alpha Blockers

♥ alfuzosin (Uroxatral)   ♥ prazosin (Minipress)
♥ doxazosin (Cardura)   ♥ terazosin (Hytrin)

The Good

Alpha-blockers are used for the treatment of high blood pressure. They lower blood pressure by blocking alpha-receptors in the smooth muscle of peripheral arteries. The alpha-receptors constrict the peripheral arteries. Blocking their action causes the peripheral arteries to relax and widen, lowering blood pressure.

Because alpha blockers also relax other muscles throughout the body, they are used in the treatment of circulatory problems such as Raynaud's disease and in the treatment of benign prostatic hyperplasia in men.

The Bad

Alpha blockers' side effects include dizziness, headache, racing heart, nausea, weakness, and weight gain.

The Ugly

Long-term use of some alpha blockers can increase the risk of heart failure. As well, some evidence suggests that using alpha blockers alone as a first-line drug choice for hypertension may actually increase the risk of heart-related problems, such as heart attacks or strokes.

The Noteworthy

When you first start taking an alpha blocker you may experience pronounced low blood pressure, which can cause dizziness and even fainting, especially when you get up from a sitting or lying down position.

Anti-Arrhythmia Drugs

♥ amiodarone (Cordarone, Pacerone)   ♥ quinidine
♥ disopyramide (Norpace)   ♥ propafenone (Rythmol)

♥ dronedarone (Multaq)
♥ flecainide (Tambocor)
♥ dofetilide (Tikosyn)
♥ procainamide (Procan, Procanbid)

♥ lidocaine (Xylocaine)
♥ ibutilide (Corvert)
♥ sotalol

Note: Some beta blockers (for example, metoprolol) and some calcium channel blockers (for example, diltiazem) are also used to treat arrhythmias.

The Good

Anti-arrhythmia drugs are used to treat abnormal heart rhythms resulting from irregular electrical activity of the heart, such as atrial fibrillation, atrial flutter, ventricular tachycardia, and ventricular fibrillation. These drugs help return the heart to its normal sinus rhythm, maintain the rhythm after it has been achieved, and/or slow the heart rate. These medicines stabilize the heart muscle tissue.

The Bad

Side effects of anti-arrhythmic drugs vary, as they each have a different mechanism of action. The most common side effects that they share are slow heartbeat, palpitations, fatigue, headache, dizziness, nausea, changes in taste or vision, difficulty breathing, and urinary retention in men. The risk of side effects is greater in those with more severe underlying heart disease.

The Ugly

Anti-arrhythmic drugs may increase the risk of developing a more severe arrhythmia (like ventricular tachycardia or ventricular fibrillation), which can be fatal. It is very important that you be closely monitored when taking these drugs.

The Noteworthy

♥ Amiodarone can be hard on every organ in the body aside from the kidneys. If you are on this drug long term, your liver, thyroid, lungs, and eyes need to be regularly examined and monitored. Signs of liver problems include abdominal pain or tenderness, dark stools or urine, fever, itching, and yellow eyes or skin. Be cautious when taking other drugs or supplements that are potentially harmful to the liver, for example, the herbs chaparral and comfrey.

♥ Amiodarone can increase a person's sensitivity to the sun, amplifying the risk of sunburn or skin rash. When outdoors, wear sunscreen with SPF 30 and protective clothing.

♥ Disopyramide can cause *hypoglycemia* (low blood sugar) in some people. It can also reduce sweating, allowing your body temperature to increase, so it is important not to become overheated during exercise when taking this medication.

Anti-Platelet Agents (Anti-Coagulants/Blood Thinners)

♥ aspirin
♥ clopidogrel (Plavix)
♥ warfarin (Coumadin)
♥ glycoprotein IIb/IIIa inhibitors (Aggrastat, ReoPro, Integrilin)
♥ unfractionated heparin
♥ low-molecular weight heparin (Enoxaparin, Dalteparin)
♥ thrombolytics (Streptokinase, tissue plasminogen activator [t-PA])

Various medications are used to thin the blood. These drugs are also known as *anti-platelet drugs* because they inhibit the ability of platelets to clump together and form a blood clot. Preventing blood clots helps to reduce the risk of a stroke or heart attack. Conditions that increase your risk of developing blood clots include *atrial fibrillation* (a certain type of irregular heart rhythm), heart valve replacement, recent heart attack, and certain surgeries such as hip or knee replacement.

Aspirin

The Good

Aspirin or *acetylsalicylic acid* (*ASA*) and other *non-steroidal anti-inflammatory drugs* (*NSAIDs*), such as ibuprofen, are commonly used to treat fever, pain, and inflammatory conditions. Aspirin also has an inhibitory effect on platelets and can prevent blood clots; it is often recommended for prevention of heart attack and stroke, particularly in those who have atherosclerosis.

Aspirin recommendations for prevention of heart disease differ for men and women. Aspirin is used for primary prevention of heart attack in men. Similar to men, women over the age of 65 should also take aspirin — but to reduce the risk of a stroke, rather than to reduce the risk of a first heart attack. In women under the age of 65, the risk of bleeding from aspirin may outweigh any benefit of reducing cardiovascular events, so it is recommended that aspirin use in this age group be considered based on risk factors, under the guidance and management of their physician. A woman of any age who has had a heart attack, coronary artery disease, or a coronary artery disease equivalent state (for example, diabetes) should be on aspirin. The usual dose recommended for primary prevention in women is 81 mg daily or 100 mg every other day.

Chewing an uncoated aspirin right away, at the first sign of chest discomfort or distress, can reduce the amount of damage to the heart muscle during a heart attack.

The Bad
Side effects of aspirin include nausea, indigestion, heartburn, and stomach ulcers.

The Ugly
Aspirin can cause serious abdominal bleeding from ulcers; this can be potentially fatal. Although aspirin is an over-the-counter drug, it should be taken only on the recommendation of a physician. Aspirin can be dangerous for people with severe liver and kidney disease, ulcers, and asthma.

The Noteworthy
- ♥ Aspirin should be taken with a full glass of water with food to reduce stomach upset.
- ♥ Alcohol should be avoided when taking aspirin because it increases the risk of stomach bleeding.
- ♥ Certain supplements can potentially enhance the blood-thinning effects of aspirin, including ginkgo biloba, garlic, and vitamin E. Talk to your doctor or pharmacist before taking any over-the-counter supplements.
- ♥ The herb white willow, which is used to treat pain and fever, contains a substance that is converted by the body into a salicylate similar to

aspirin. It is therefore possible that taking aspirin and white willow could lead to increased risk of side effects.

♥ Taking other drugs containing aspirin or NSAIDs may increase the risk of bleeding, so be cautious when choosing over-the-counter cold remedies and pain relievers, as many of them contain aspirin.

♥ If you are planning to have surgery or a dental procedure, discuss with your doctor if it is really safe to stop aspirin, even for a short time. Many diagnostic or surgical procedures can be safely performed while on low doses of aspirin.

♥ Aspirin can deplete various nutrients in the body, including folic acid, iron, potassium, and vitamin C. Offset these depletions by supplementing with a quality multivitamin. Ask your doctor or pharmacist for a recommendation.

> *Research suggests that when heart attack or stroke survivors who are prescribed daily aspirin stop taking the drug, they may triple their risk of having another stroke within days. If you are taking aspirin for heart attack or stroke prevention, check with your doctor before you stop taking it for any reason.*

Clopidogrel (Plavix)

The Good
Clopidogrel is prescribed to prevent heart attacks and strokes in people with heart disease (recent heart attack, unstable angina), recent stroke, or blood circulation disease (peripheral vascular disease). It is particularly prescribed to those who are allergic to or experience side effects with aspirin. In some cases it is given along with aspirin.

The Bad
Side effects of clopidogrel include upset stomach, increased bruising, diarrhea, constipation, dizziness, heartburn, headache, rash, and itching.

The Ugly
Stomach and intestinal bleeding can occur with clopidogrel, although it is less common than with aspirin. Contact your doctor immediately if

you experience any signs of serious bleeding: unusual or easy bruising, bleeding that won't stop, black stools, or vomit that looks like coffee grounds. Other rare but serious side effects include a reduction in white blood cell count and a condition called *thrombotic thrombocytopenic purpura*, which is the formation of blood clots throughout the body.

The Noteworthy
♥ Before having surgery, tell your doctor or dentist that you are taking this medication. Your doctor may instruct you to stop clopidogrel prior to surgery. However, do not stop taking clopidogrel unless advised to do so by your doctor. Suddenly stopping this medication may increase the risk of a heart attack.
♥ Limit alcoholic beverages. Daily use of alcohol, especially when combined with this medicine, may increase your risk for stomach bleeding.
♥ Taking clopidogrel along with non-steroidal anti-inflammatory drugs (NSAIDs) such as ibuprofen (Motrin, Advil) may increase the risk of stomach and intestinal bleeding.
♥ Various herbs and supplements might interfere with the ability of the blood to clot. If they are taken with clopidogrel, excess bleeding might occur; see the list of possible interactions noted in the warfarin section below.

Warfarin (Coumadin)

The Good
Warfarin is prescribed to treat blood clots and/or to prevent new clots from forming. It works by decreasing the amount of clotting proteins in the blood.

The Bad
Common side effects of warfarin include nausea, loss of appetite, and stomach pain.

The Ugly
Warfarin can cause serious, life-threatening bleeding. Even if you stop taking the drug, the risk of bleeding can continue for up to a week afterwards. If you are taking warfarin, be aware of the signs of

serious bleeding, including unusual pain; swelling or discomfort; easy bruising; prolonged bleeding from cuts; bleeding gums; persistent or frequent nosebleeds; unusually heavy or prolonged menstrual flow; pink or dark urine; coughing up blood; vomit that is bloody or looks like coffee grounds; severe headache; dizziness or fainting; unusual or persistent tiredness or weakness; bloody, black, or tarry stools; chest pain; shortness of breath; or difficulty swallowing.

The Noteworthy

♥ Warfarin should be taken at the same time every day, preferably at night. It can be taken without food.

♥ Many drugs and supplements interact with warfarin. Supplements that can reduce the action of warfarin include alfalfa, St. John's wort, coenzyme Q10, and vitamin K. Supplements that have blood-thinning effects and can enhance the action of warfarin include garlic, ginger, ginkgo biloba, policosanol, vitamin E, and white willow. Always check with your pharmacist before taking any new drug, over-the-counter product, or supplement.

♥ Consuming large amounts of foods high in vitamin K (such as broccoli, spinach, and other green, leafy vegetables) may reduce the effect of warfarin. It is okay to eat these foods, but try to keep the amount of these foods in your diet consistent.

♥ Don't drink alcohol while taking warfarin, as it can reduce the drug's efficacy.

♥ To reduce the chance of gum bleeding, use a soft toothbrush and floss gently. Be cautious using razors. If you are having surgery or dental work, you may need to stop taking warfarin for a few days beforehand. But check with the doctor who prescribed you warfarin before stopping it.

♥ Your doctor will order frequent blood tests when you first start the drug to determine the correct dose of warfarin for you. The *prothrombin time* (PT) test is used to calculate your *international normalized ratio* (INR). Your INR will help your doctor determine how fast your blood is clotting and whether your medication dose needs to be changed. Once your therapeutic dosage has been established, your blood will be checked less frequently (possibly monthly). If you start taking certain drugs or supplements your doctor may need to order more frequent INR levels.

Certain anti-platelet drugs are given by injection in the hospital or, in the case of low-molecular weight heparin, as part of outpatient treatment once your condition is stabilized. Here is a brief description of each.

Glycoprotein IIb/IIIa Inhibitors

Glycoprotein IIb/IIIa inhibitors are classified as potent *platelet inhibitors* (they prevent platelets from binding together). These drugs are used to treat unstable angina, certain types of heart attacks, and are used in combination with angioplasty with or without stent placement. They are also given in combination with heparin or aspirin to prevent clotting before and during invasive heart procedures.

Unfractionated heparin

Unfractionated Heparin is used to prevent blood clots from forming in people who have certain medical conditions (such as pulmonary embolism, deep vein thrombosis, and atrial fibrillation with embolism) or who are undergoing certain medical procedures that increase the chance of blood clots. It works by decreasing the clotting ability of the blood.

Unfractionated heparin is also used to stop the growth of clots that have already formed in the blood vessels, but it cannot be used to decrease the size of clots that have already formed.

Low-molecular weight heparin (LMWH)

LMWH is similar to regular heparin but consists of smaller chains of molecules with a lower weight, hence the name. These drugs are given subcutaneously (under the skin), thus they are more suitable for outpatient treatment of conditions such as deep vein thrombosis and pulmonary embolism that is stabilized.

Studies show women who are eligible candidates to receive life-saving clot-buster drugs are far less likely than men to receive them. In a study from Washington state, only 55 percent of eligible women with heart attack received thrombolytic drugs compared with 78 percent of men.

Thrombolytics

Thrombolytic drugs are used to break up or dissolve blood clots, which are the main cause of both heart attacks and stroke. The most commonly used thrombolytic is tissue plasminogen activator (tPA); other drugs in this class are streptokinase and urokinase. According to the American Heart Association, you have a better chance of surviving and recovering from a heart attack if you receive a thrombolytic drug within 12 hours after the heart attack starts. Ideally, you should receive thrombolytic medications within the first 90 minutes after arriving at the hospital for treatment. Having thrombolytics within three hours of the first stroke symptoms can help limit stroke damage and disability.

Note: All anti-platelet drugs, including ASA, carry the risk of bleeding. Women may have more bleeding when taking these drugs. The reason for this is unknown.

Women treated with clot-busting drugs during a heart attack fare better than women who do not receive these drugs. In an overview of nine research studies, clot-busting medications reduced the risk of a woman dying within 35 days after a heart attack by 12 percent.

ARBs (Angiotensin II Receptor Blockers)

♥ candesartan (Atacand) ♥ telmisartan (Micardis)
♥ irbesartan (Avapro) ♥ valsartan (Diovan)
♥ losartan (Cozaar)

The Good

ARBs have the same effects on heart disease as ACE inhibitors but work by a different mechanism. They act to decrease chemicals that narrow the blood vessels, allowing blood to flow more easily through the body. They also reduce chemicals that cause salt and fluid buildup in the body.

ARBs are prescribed for the same reasons as ACE inhibitors: to treat high blood pressure and heart failure and to prevent heart attack and stroke in those at high risk. ARBs are most often used by people who have experienced side effects with ACE inhibitors.

The Bad
The most common side effects of ARBs are dizziness, lightheadedness, headache, diarrhea, elevated potassium levels (*hyperkalemia*), change in taste, muscle cramps, and respiratory infection.

The Ugly
The most serious, but rare, side effects of ARBs are kidney or liver failure, decreased white blood cells, and swelling of tissues (*angioedema*).

The Noteworthy
♥ Avoid using salt substitutes when taking an ARB. Salt substitutes contain potassium and ARBs cause the body to retain potassium.
♥ Over-the-counter non-steroidal anti-inflammatory medications (such as Motrin or Advil) and aspirin may cause the body to retain salt and water and decrease the efficacy of an ACE inhibitor. Check with your doctor or pharmacist before taking any anti-inflammatory medications or other over-the-counter medications or supplements.
♥ Many of these medications are not recommended for women who are pregnant or breastfeeding. Check with your doctor if you are pregnant, plan to get pregnant, or are breastfeeding.
♥ While taking an ARB, have your blood pressure and kidney function checked regularly, as recommended by your doctor.

Beta Blockers
♥ acebutolol (Sectral)
♥ atenolol (Tenormin)
♥ bisoprolol (Zebeta, Monocor)
♥ carvedilol (Coreg, Coreg-CR)
♥ esmolol (Brevibloc)
♥ labetolol (Trandate, Normodyne)
♥ metoprolol (Lopressor, Toprol XL)
♥ nebivolol (Bystolic)
♥ propranolol (Inderal)
♥ sotalol (Betapace, Sotalex, Sotacor)

The Good
Beta blockers are prescribed for managing symptoms of heart disease, high blood pressure, arrhythmias, angina, and heart failure. They are often given after a heart attack to prevent further heart attacks and death.

Beta blockers slow the heart rate and reduce the force with which the heart muscle contracts, thereby lowering blood pressure. They achieve this by blocking beta-adrenergic receptors, which prevents adrenaline (*epinephrine*) from stimulating these receptors. Over time, beta blockers improve the heart's pumping ability.

The Bad

Common side effects of beta blockers include dizziness, fatigue, constipation, diarrhea, nausea, vomiting, slow heart rate, impotence, decreased libido, weight gain, and trouble sleeping. Less common side effects include dry and sore eyes; swelling of ankles, feet and lower legs; cold hands and feet; itchy skin or skin rash; frequent urination; unusual bleeding and bruising; hallucinations; fever; and sore throat. Elderly people tend to be more sensitive to the side effects, particularly cold hands and feet.

The Ugly

Rare but more concerning side effects include difficulty breathing, depression, anxiety, and confusion.

The Noteworthy

♥ Beta blockers can mask signs of low blood sugar in people with diabetes. They can also aggravate asthma.

♥ Use of beta blockers during pregnancy may cause slowed heart rate, low blood sugar, and low blood pressure in the baby. These drugs can also slow the flow of breast milk and can be passed on to babies through breast milk. Nonetheless, some beta blockers can be used during pregnancy.

♥ Beta blockers slow the heart rate, even during exercise. This means that your heart rate may not increase past a certain point no matter how hard you are working out. Thus, monitoring your heart rate during exercise will not give you an accurate indication of the intensity of your workout.

♥ Beta blockers can reduce tolerance to exercise, meaning that your heart may not be able to supply your body's increased demands for blood and oxygen, reducing your overall endurance.

♥ Beta blockers (particularly metoprolol and propranolol) can deplete the body's levels of coenzyme Q10 (CoQ10), an important nutrient for heart health (see Chapter 7). CoQ10 is an antioxidant that plays a critical role in cellular energy production. Depletion of CoQ10 might be responsible for some of the side effects of beta blockers. Supplementing with CoQ10 can correct this depletion and possibly offset side effects.

Calcium Channel Blockers

♥ amlodipine (Norvasc)   ♥ diltiazem (Cardizem, Tiazac)
♥ felodipine (Plendil)   ♥ isradipine (Dynacirc)
♥ nicardipine (Cardene)   ♥ nifedipine (Adalat, Procardia)
♥ nimodipine (Nimotop)   ♥ nisoldipine (Sular)
♥ verapamil (Calan, Isoptin)

The Good

Calcium channel blockers relax blood vessels and increase the supply of blood and oxygen to the heart by reducing the amount of work the heart must do to pump blood to the body. These medications are used to treat coronary heart disease, angina, arrhythmias, and high blood pressure.

The Bad

Side effects of calcium channel blockers include fatigue, dizziness, lightheadedness, headache, increased appetite, nausea, diarrhea, con-stipation, heartburn, swelling of the ankles and legs, slow heart rate, flushing, and nasal congestion.

The Ugly

If you experience shortness of breath, coughing, sudden weight gain, or tenderness or bleeding of the gums, call your doctor right away. These are signs of intolerance to the drug or worsening of the condi-tion where calcium channel blockers should not be used.

The Noteworthy

♥ Do not eat grapefruit or drink grapefruit juice while taking a cal-cium channel blocker. Grapefruit contains compounds that reduce how the drug is metabolized, leading to higher than normal drug levels in the body. This occurs most prominently with felodipine.
♥ Taking calcium or vitamin D supplements may interfere with some of the effects of calcium channel blockers. Consult your doctor before taking these supplements.

♥ Avoid alcohol, as it interferes with the effects of calcium channel blockers and increases the risk of side effects.

♥ Consult your doctor before taking calcium channel blockers during pregnancy. Animal studies suggest that some calcium channel blockers may cause birth defects and even stillbirth.

Cholesterol-Lowering Medications

♥ bile acid sequestrants   ♥ cholesterol absorption inhibitors
♥ fibrates   ♥ nicotinic acid
♥ omega-3 fatty acids   ♥ statins

Certain medications can lower levels of LDL (bad) cholesterol and triglycerides (blood fats) and increase blood levels of desirable lipids such as HDL (good) cholesterol. (We told you more about the different types of cholesterol in Chapter 2.) Several classes of medications are available, including statins (HMG CoA reductase inhibitors), fibrates, bile acid sequestrants, and cholesterol absorption inhibitors. These drug classes are discussed below. Nicotinic acid (niacin, or vitamin B3), and omega-3 fatty acids (found in fish oils) are available as nutritional supplements and as prescription drugs, so they are discussed briefly here; you can read more about them in Chapter 7.

Depending on your lipid profile, your doctor may prescribe more than one medication to more aggressively manage your condition.

Bile Acid Sequestrants (Resins)

♥ cholestyramine (Questran, Questran Light, Prevalite, Locholest, Locholest Light)
♥ colesevelam (Welchol)
♥ colestipol (Colestid)

The Good

Bile acid sequestrants are used to lower LDL cholesterol. Because they have modest effects compared with other drugs, they are often used in combination with a statin or with niacin (which we discuss a bit later on in this chapter) to enhance the LDL cholesterol–lowering effects of those drugs. Bile acid sequestrants work by binding to bile acids in the intestine and promoting their elimination in the stool. This reduces the amount of bile acids returning to the liver and forces the liver to produce more bile acids. To do this, the liver converts cholesterol into bile acids, which lowers the level of cholesterol in the blood.

The Bad
The most common side effects of bile acid sequestrants are constipation, abdominal pain, gas, bloating, vomiting, diarrhea, and weight loss.

The Ugly
There are reports of bile acid sequestrants increasing risk of gallstones because of increased cholesterol concentration in the bile.

The Noteworthy
♥ Long-term use of cholestyramine may cause a deficiency of vitamins A, D, E, and K because bile acid sequestrants reduce the absorption of these vitamins.
♥ Calcium, iron, and folate may also be depleted. Long-term use may thus cause a deficiency of these nutrients.
♥ Bile acid sequestrants can bind to and decrease the absorption (and effectiveness) of other drugs and supplements, so take other medications or supplements one hour before or four to six hours after taking a bile acid sequestrant.

Cholesterol Absorption Inhibitors
♥ ezetimibe (Zetia in the United States; Ezetrol in Canada)

The Good
Cholesterol absorption inhibitors make up a fairly new class of cholesterol-lowering medications. They work by blocking the absorption of cholesterol, including dietary cholesterol, from the intestines. The only drug available so far in this class is ezetimibe. It is most effective at lowering LDL (bad) cholesterol but may also have modest effects on lowering triglycerides and raising HDL (good) cholesterol levels.

The Bad
The most common side effects of cholesterol absorption inhibitors are diarrhea, headache, abdominal pain, back pain, joint pain, and sinusitis.

The Ugly
Pancreatitis, muscle damage (*myopathy* or *rhabdomyolysis*), and hepatitis have also been reported with this drug.

The Noteworthy

Ezetimibe is often combined with a low-dose statin to boost efficacy and prevent the need for higher-dose statin therapy. When used together these drugs are more effective in improving cholesterol and triglyceride levels than either treatment alone.

Fibrates

- ♥ clofibrate (Atromid-S)
- ♥ fenofibrate (Lipidil and Lipidil Micro in Canada; Tricor in the United States)
- ♥ fenofibric acid (Trilipix)
- ♥ gemfibrozil (Lopid)

The Good

Fibrates are used primarily to lower triglycerides. They work by inhibiting the liver's production of *VLDL* (particles in the blood that carry triglycerides and lipoproteins) and speeding up the removal of triglycerides from the blood. They have a modest effect on increasing HDL (good) cholesterol levels but are not effective in lowering LDL (bad) cholesterol levels. For this reason they are sometimes combined with statins.

The Bad

Common side effects of fibrates include upset stomach, constipation or diarrhea, headache, and dizziness.

The Ugly

Fibrates can cause muscle damage. This risk is higher when these drugs are used with statins. Any muscle pain or weakness should be reported to your doctor immediately. Fibrates can also cause liver irritation, which is usually mild and reversible. Signs may include yellowing of the eyes or skin (*jaundice*) and abdominal pain.

The Noteworthy

- ♥ Fibrates can increase the blood-thinning effect of drugs like warfarin (see our earlier discussion of warfarin in this chapter). Taking supplements that also thin the blood, like ginkgo biloba and vitamin E, can potentially intensify this effect.

Nicotinic Acid
♥ niacin (sold off the shelf in health food stores and pharmacies)
♥ Niaspan (prescription form of nicotinic acid)

The Good
Nicotinic acid can significantly lower triglycerides and raise HDL cholesterol. It also helps lower LDL cholesterol, but to a lesser extent, and it decreases levels of lipoprotein(a) and fibrinogen. Several studies have looked at the effects of niacin, alone and in combination with other drugs, for the prevention of heart disease and fatal heart attacks. Overall, this research suggests benefits of niacin, especially when combined with other cholesterol-lowering drugs.

The Bad
Side effects include headache, skin itching and rash, and flushing. Nicotinic acid can increase homocysteine levels and elevated homocysteine can have a negative impact on heart health. (Chapter 2 provides more information about homocysteine.)

The Ugly
Nicotinic acid can cause elevated liver enzymes and liver inflammation; when it is taken with statins there is a risk of *rhabdomyolysis*, a condition in which muscle cells are broken down, releasing enzymes into the blood and potentially causing kidney failure. Use of niacin requires close monitoring by your doctor.

The Noteworthy
♥ Nicotinic acid can increase the risk of gout and may worsen diabetes.
♥ If you experience flushing while taking niacin, see Chapter 7 for tips on how to reduce this side effect.
♥ Taking "no-flush" niacin (inositol hexaniacinate) does not offer the same benefits: what causes the flushing is what makes this product effective at improving your cholesterol.

Omega-3 Fatty Acids
♥ Prescription drug known as Lovaza (in the U.S.) or Omacor (in all other countries)
♥ Supplemental (off-the-shelf) fish oil

The Good

The omega-3 fatty acids *eicosapentaenoic acid* (EPA) and *docosa-hexaenoic acid* (DHA) offer a number of benefits for the heart. They reduce inflammation and clotting, significantly lower triglycerides, and modestly raise HDL cholesterol. These beneficial fats may also help reduce blood pressure, lower levels of homocysteine, and improve blood vessel tone. Studies have also shown that they can reduce the risk of sudden cardiac death and arrhythmias.

The Bad

Side effects include belching (fishy odor), upset stomach, rash, and change in taste.

The Ugly

High doses of omega-3 fatty acids (4 grams daily) can significantly raise LDL cholesterol levels — by as much as 49%. But if the primary reason for taking them is to reduce your triglyceride levels, your doctor may keep you on them and also prescribe another medication to keep your LDL in control.

The Noteworthy

♥ Supplemental fish oils are not equivalent to prescription fish oil (Lovaza/Omacor); they contain lower amounts of DHA and EPA, may have increased mercury and toxins, and contain more saturated fats.

♥ High doses of omega-3 fatty acids can increase the risk of bleeding in some people. You should stop taking these products before having surgery.

Statins

♥ atorvastatin (Lipitor)	♥ fluvastatin (Lescol)
♥ lovastatin (Mevacor)	♥ pravastatin (Pravachol)
♥ rosuvastatin (Crestor)	♥ simvastatin (Zocor)

The Good

Statins are the most widely used medications for lowering LDL (bad) cholesterol. They also modestly decrease triglycerides and raise HDL cholesterol. These drugs work by reducing the production of cholesterol by the liver. Specifically, they block the enzyme in the liver (*HMG-CoA reductase*) that controls the production of cholesterol. Statins are prescribed for those with high cholesterol. They are also used for treating and preventing atherosclerosis in the heart arteries, in addition to other arteries in the circulatory system. Numerous studies have shown that statins reduce heart attacks and strokes and improve survival rates.

The Bad
Side effects of statins include constipation, diarrhea, fatigue, gas, heartburn, headache, and muscle pain.

The Ugly
Statin drugs can elevate liver enzymes and in serious, but rare cases can cause liver failure and *rhabdomyolysis* (muscle inflammation and breakdown). Symptoms of rhabdomyolysis include muscle pain, weakness, tenderness, fever, dark urine, nausea, and vomiting. In severe cases, rhabdomyolysis can result in kidney failure and can be life-threatening.

The Noteworthy
♥ St. John's wort may decrease blood levels of various statins, particularly atorvastatin, lovastatin, and simvastatin.

♥ Grapefruit juice interferes with enzymes that are responsible for breaking down several drugs, including statins, allowing them to build up to excessive levels in the blood. This can be potentially dangerous, increasing the risk of liver and kidney damage. The statins most affected are atorvastatin, lovastatin, and simvastatin. It is best to avoid grapefruit juice altogether when taking these statins. Grapefruit juice may not affect rosuvastatin, fluvastatin, or pravastatin because these drugs are broken down by different enzymes.

♥ Combining niacin, which is available over-the-counter and also used for lowering cholesterol, with statins can increase the risk of *rhabdomyolysis* (muscle inflammation and breakdown). This combination should be used only under doctor supervision.

♥ Red yeast rice, a natural product used for lowering cholesterol, contains a statin component, lovastatin; thus combining it with statins could increase the risk of side effects.

♥ Statins can deplete levels of coenzyme Q10, an antioxidant that is important for heart function and energy production in the body (see Chapter 7). CoQ10 deficiency may impair heart function and increase the risk of statin side effects, including muscle weakness.

♥ Some, but not all, studies have shown that supplementing with CoQ10 can improve muscle weakness and pain caused by statins.

Digoxin
♥ digoxin (Lanoxin, Lanoxicaps)

The Good
Digoxin helps the heart work more efficiently. It strengthens the force of the heart muscle's contractions and slows the heart rate. This leads to better blood circulation and reduced swelling of the hands and ankles in people with heart problems. Digoxin is prescribed for heart failure and atrial fibrillation.

The Bad
Side effects of digoxin include loss of appetite, nausea, vomiting, drowsiness, headache, confusion, depression, fatigue, muscle weakness, and changes in vision such as flashes or flickering of light, sensitivity to light, blurring, color changes (yellow or green), and seeing halos on objects. These side effects may go away with time as your body adjusts to the medication.

The Van Gogh effect
The noted ocular side effect of digoxin toxicity is typified by generalized blurry vision as well as seeing a "halo" around lights. This effect is best exemplified by Vincent van Gogh's painting "Starry Night," in which there is a halo effect around each star in the sky. Evidence supporting van Gogh's digoxin use is the multiple self-portraits that include the foxglove plant, from which digoxin is obtained.

The Ugly
If you experience any of the following side effects, contact your doctor immediately: dizziness; fainting; fast, pounding, or irregular heartbeat or pulse; slow heartbeat; severe stomach pain; or unusual bleeding. These side effects could mean that your dosage is too high and needs to be adjusted.

The Noteworthy
- ♥ Digoxin works best when there is a constant amount in the blood, so take it at the same time each day.
- ♥ While you're taking this medication, your doctor may tell you to take and record your pulse daily. If your pulse is too high or too low, call your doctor before you take your next dose.
- ♥ Digoxin is excreted by the kidneys; if your kidney function worsens, your dosage will need to be reduced.
- ♥ Magnesium deficiency can increase the risk of toxicity from digoxin. Magnesium supplements can be taken under your doctor's advice, but it is important to separate the time that you take magnesium and the time you take digoxin by two hours, as it can impair the body's absorption of digoxin.
- ♥ Licorice root can lower potassium levels in the body, which can be dangerous if you are taking digoxin.
- ♥ St. John's wort may interact with digoxin, possibly requiring an increased dosage to maintain the proper effect.

Diuretics
Loop diuretics:
- ♥ bumetanide (Bumex)
- ♥ furosemide (Lasix)

Potassium-sparing diuretics:
- ♥ amiloride (Moduret in Canada, Benzamil in the United States)
- ♥ eplerenone (Inspra)
- ♥ spironolactone (Aldactone)

Thiazide diuretics:
- ♥ hydrochlorothiazide (Hydrodiuril)
- ♥ metolazone (Zytanix, Zaroxolyn, Mykrox)

The Good
Also known as "water pills," *diuretics* help your body eliminate excess water and salt through the urine. This makes it easier for your heart to pump and control blood pressure. These drugs are prescribed for the management of heart failure, to reduce swelling (*edema*) that often occurs in the legs, and also to prevent fluid buildup in the lungs. They are also used for the treatment of high blood pressure, kidney and liver disease, and glaucoma.

There are three main classes of diuretics; each works differently:

♥ *Loop diuretics* inhibit the kidneys' ability to reabsorb sodium, thus enhancing the loss of sodium in the urine. And when sodium is lost in the urine, water goes with it.

♥ *Potassium-sparing diuretics* help eliminate water by blocking the exchange of sodium for potassium, resulting in excretion of sodium and potassium, but relatively little loss of potassium. Eplerenone and spironolactone, which were discussed earlier, work by blocking aldosterones. Amiloride blocks the sodium channel, thereby reducing sodium reabsorption.

♥ *Thiazide diuretics* enhance the excretion of both sodium and chloride in the urine so that water is eliminated from the body.

The Bad

The most common side effects of diuretics include frequent urination (as this is how the drug works to remove excess fluid), weakness, headache, low blood pressure, dehydration, thirst, muscle cramps, change in electrolyte balance, dizziness, skin rash, nausea, and vomiting.

The Ugly

Imbalances in fluids and electrolytes (low sodium, low magnesium, and high potassium) may occur and can be harmful to the heart and the kidneys. This is why regular monitoring is important when taking a diuretic. Spironolactone can cause enlargement of the breasts (*gynecomastia*); this usually goes away when the medication is stopped.

The Noteworthy

♥ If you are taking a single daily dose, take it in the morning with your breakfast to avoid late-night trips to the bathroom. If you are taking more than one dose a day, take the last dose no later than 4 p.m.

♥ If you are taking a loop or thiazide diuretic, your doctor may recommend a potassium supplement or increasing your intake of potassium-rich foods such as bananas and oranges. These diuretics can also cause magnesium deficiency, which can lead to muscle cramps and weakness. Supplementing with magnesium may be necessary.

♥ If you are taking a potassium-sparing diuretic, it is not advisable to take potassium supplements because your potassium levels might rise too high.

♥ Loop diuretics can cause increased sensitivity to the sun, increasing the risk of sunburn or skin rash. The herbs St. John's wort and dong quai can also cause sun sensitivity. Taking these herbs with a loop diuretic may increase the risk of sunburn, so wear protective clothing and sunscreen when outdoors.

Nitroglycerin
♥ nitroglycerin (Nitrolingual, Nitro-Dur, Nitrostat, Nitrotab)

The Good
Nitroglycerin belongs to a class of drugs called *nitrates*. These drugs relax and dilate the blood vessels (arteries and veins), increasing the supply of blood and oxygen to the heart and reducing the workload on the heart. Nitrates are prescribed for the management of heart pain (*angina*) in those with heart disease.

Nitroglycerin is available in several forms: sublingual tablets, capsules, spray, ointment, and patches. The capsules, patches, and ointment are used daily to prevent angina attacks, and the oral spray and sublingual tablets are used to halt an angina attack that has already started.

The Bad
Side effects of nitroglycerin include headache, flushing, sweating, dizziness, and nausea.

The Ugly
Nitroglycerin can cause an increase in heart rate, heart palpitations, and a drop in blood pressure, which can cause dizziness and fainting. To reduce the risk of low blood pressure and fainting, sit or lie down during and immediately after taking nitroglycerin.

The Noteworthy
♥ Alcoholic beverages may increase the risk of fainting or of experiencing dizziness.
♥ Symptoms of overdose include a persistent, throbbing headache; dizziness; confusion; weakness; sweating; changes in heart rate; changes in vision; flushing; nausea; and vomiting.
♥ Nitroglycerin sublingual tablets should not be chewed, crushed, or swallowed. They are absorbed more quickly and work faster when placed under the tongue to dissolve.

♥ Vitamin C may help prevent developing a tolerance to nitrate medications. Studies show that it also helps maintain the effectiveness of nitroglycerine. Consult with your pharmacist for advice on taking vitamin C supplements.

Renin Inhibitors
♥ aliskiren (Tekturna)

The Good
Renin inhibitors block the enzyme renin from triggering a process that tightens blood vessels. As a result, blood vessels relax and widen, lowering blood pressure and allowing the heart to pump blood more efficiently. These drugs are used alone or in combination with a diuretic (see the section on "Diuretics") or other drugs for treating high blood pressure (*hypertension*).

The Bad
The most common side effects are diarrhea, heartburn, and stomach pain.

The Ugly
There are no serious or life-threatening side effects of this drug unless you are allergic to it.

This drug is not recommended for use during pregnancy, as it may cause serious and potentially fatal harm to an unborn baby.

The Noteworthy
This is the newest drug class to emerge recently, and to date no data exists to support that renin inhibitors improve outcomes when used after a heart attack.

Vasodilators
Alpha2 Agonists
♥ clonidine (Catapres)   ♥ guanabenz (Wytensin)
♥ guanfacine (Tenex)   ♥ methyldopa (Aldomet and Aldoril)
Hydralazine (Apresoline)

The Good

Alpha2 agonists are also known as *centrally acting* drugs. They stimulate alpha-receptors in the brain, which causes the peripheral arteries to relax (dilate), thereby lowering both blood pressure and heart rate.

Hydralazine is another vasodilator, but its mechanism of action is not fully known, putting it in a class by itself. It is used in both hypertension and in heart failure. It works to relax the smooth muscles in the arteries and arterioles, making it useful for treating hypertension. It also increases both heart rate and cardiac output (increasing the amount of blood the heart can pump to the body), making it useful in those with heart failure.

The Bad

Side effects of alpha2 agonists include extreme fatigue, drowsiness, dizziness, headache, constipation, dry mouth, weight gain, impaired thinking, and impotence in men.

Side effects of hydralazine include headache, nausea, vomiting, diarrhea, palpitations, racing heart, fluid retention, and angina.

The Ugly

Abruptly stopping these drugs can cause a sudden and dangerous increase in blood pressure. Hydralazine can cause heart attack in some individuals.

The Noteworthy

♥ There is some evidence that clonidine and methyldopa might impair the body's ability to manufacture the antioxidant coenzyme Q10; taking supplements can help offset this depletion.

♥ Methyldopa, alone or in combination with hydralazine, can be safely used during pregnancy.

Managing Your Medication

It is important to know how to benefit the most from any heart medication you have been prescribed, and how to reduce your risk of problems. Keep these tips in mind when managing your medication:

♥ When prescribed a new medication, ask how it should be taken (time of day, with or without meals) and if there are any side effects, precautions, or interactions with your other medications.

♥ Take your medication exactly as prescribed. There are reasons why certain drugs are best taken in the morning or evening. Changing the time that you take your medications or the amount could lead to side effects and health risks. Don't change or stop taking your medications unless advised by your doctor, as this could worsen your condition.

♥ If you forget to take a dose, take it as soon as you remember. However, if it is almost time for your next dose, ask your doctor or pharmacist about whether you should skip or make up the missed dose.

♥ Get your prescriptions refilled a few days before you run out so that you don't risk being stuck without medication. Some pharmacies offer medication refill reminders — for example, automated phone calls or computer-generated mail-outs.

♥ Carry a list of your medications with you. It is important to know the names of your medications, the dosages, and what they are for (e.g., blood pressure or cholesterol). Keep this list in your wallet. Should you be taken to the hospital, this information will be helpful to the doctors and nurses.

♥ If you are taking multiple medications, ask your pharmacist to help you make a chart noting the times to take each medication. Pillboxes (dosettes) can be used to organize your medications and help you remember when to take them. They are available with daily, weekly, and monthly compartments.

♥ If you are purchasing an over-the-counter drug or supplement, ask your pharmacist if there are any potential interactions (good or bad) with the medications you are taking.

♥ Before having surgery or dental work, inform your surgeon or dentist of all medications (prescription and over-the-counter) that you are taking. Some drugs and supplements can increase the risk of bleeding and need to be discontinued a few days before surgery.

♥ If you are taking a trip, bring extra medication with you in case your trip is extended for some reason. It is also important to keep your medication with you (in a carry-on bag rather than checked luggage).

♥ See your doctor regularly to have your blood pressure and heart rate checked and for other routine monitoring.

The Heart of the Matter

It is important to be an informed patient — to understand the benefits and risks of your medication and how to take it properly. You'll learn in the next chapter which medications are considered standard of care for your condition. As we point out throughout the book, differences exist in how men and women are treated when it comes to heart disease. Don't be afraid to discuss any concerns you have with your doctor. Ultimately, though, knowing which medications and other measures will give you the best outcomes will empower you on the road to better heart health.

Chapter 6

Therapeutic Options and Treatment Goals for Heart Disease and Specific Cardiac Risk Factors

You only live once, but if you do it right, once is enough.
— Mae West

In this chapter, you'll learn about treatment options for certain cardiovascular conditions and heart disease risk factors. Treatment is often composed of both medication and lifestyle changes: medications alone are not enough. We'll also tell you which medications are necessary for specific conditions — those that can prolong your life, improve your condition, or reduce the risk of having a heart attack or stroke in the future — and we'll outline the goals of treatment.

For more about specific medications, refer back to Chapter 5; and be sure to read the later chapters of this book for more details about making important lifestyle changes that will benefit your heart.

Cardiovascular Conditions
Coronary Artery Disease (CAD)
Definition: The narrowing of one or more coronary arteries; also called coronary heart disease.

Therapeutic Options

The goal of any therapy given after the diagnosis of coronary artery disease is to reduce the risk of a future heart attack and other heart-related conditions. Making therapeutic lifestyle changes and taking the right medications are both important parts of reducing your risks.

Lifestyle Changes

♥ Smoking: Quit smoking; this lifestyle change is essential to reducing your risk for a heart attack or stroke.

♥ Diet: Eat a heart-healthy diet (lots of fruits and vegetables, fiber, whole grains, lean meats, and omega-3–rich fish twice a week) and reduce your intake of sugar and simple carbohydrates. Limit your alcohol intake to less than one drink (5 ounces of wine) a day. (More heart-smart nutrition information is available in Chapter 8.)

♥ Exercise: Get regular, moderately intense exercise at least 30 minutes a day (or more if you are trying to lose weight). (See Chapter 9 for more on exercise and your heart.)

♥ Weight control: Work toward achieving and maintaining a healthy body weight if you are obese or overweight.

♥ Stress control: Reduce high stress levels, which can increase your risk of a heart attack. See Chapter 10 for more on the effects of stress and what you can do to reduce it.

> Women's hearts respond better than men's to healthy lifestyle changes, yet only 2% of the National Institutes of Health's budget is dedicated to prevention.

Medications

♥ Aspirin and anti-platelet agents: Unless a doctor advises otherwise, everyone with CAD should be on aspirin, as aspirin can prevent future heart attacks, unless another health concern exists that makes taking aspirin inadvisable. Speak to your doctor about what is right for you. Clopidogrel (Plavix), an anti-platelet agent, may be given during a heart attack (see below) and after a coronary artery stent is placed (for at least one year, but usually indefinitely).

♥ Beta blockers: Beta blockers slow the heart rate down and help the blood vessels relax. In addition to their beneficial effects on the heart and blood pressure, beta blockers are proven to reduce the risk of future heart attacks and sudden cardiac death.

♥ ACE-inhibitors: These drugs, which inhibit the normal formation of the hormone that causes the blood vessels to narrow (*angiotensin II*) can reduce the risk of heart attack and stroke and improve your chances of survival. You may be prescribed an *angiotensin II receptor blocker* (ARB) if your body cannot tolerate an ACE-inhibitor.

♥ Statins: Everyone with CAD should be on a statin (drugs typically prescribed to lower blood cholesterol), as their other properties reduce the risk of a future heart attack or stroke and improve survival.[1,2,3]

♥ Nitrates: These are useful to relieve symptoms that can persist with chronic CAD, but nitrates do not affect survival.

♥ Omega-3 fatty acids: For heart attack survivors, using omega-3 fatty acids has proven benefits. In one study, participants who were given 1 gram of fish oil a day showed significant improvement in survival after just three months, compared to participants who had also had a heart attack but were given a placebo. Particularly reduced was the risk of sudden cardiac death.[4] In the United States, there is only one prescription omega-3, called Lovaza. It is the purest form available, but it is expensive and not available everywhere. Ask your doctor to recommend an omega-3 supplement that is right for you.

♥ Medications to control cardiac risk factors: If you have any factors that put you at risk for CAD (including high blood pressure, high cholesterol, and diabetes), it is important to control them. Discuss with your doctor what medication you need to do this.

♥ Annual flu vaccine and one-time pneumococcal vaccine: These vaccinations are beneficial for those with CAD, because they can prevent you from getting a severe illness — any severe illness can be stressful for the heart.

Women undergo fewer heart disease procedures than men; however, more is not necessarily better. Research has yet to establish the best course of treatment for a woman with heart disease.

Treatment Goals

If you have or are at risk of developing coronary artery disease, the goal of your treatment is to protect your heart and reduce the risk of further damaging your heart because of a heart attack (or subsequent heart attack if you have already suffered one) or other cardiovascular events, and also to reduce your risk of a stroke. Working to reduce your risk takes a combination of therapeutic lifestyle changes and lifelong medications.

Heart Attack

Definition: A sudden interruption of the blood supply to the heart muscle.

Therapeutic Options

The immediate response to a heart attack requires proven, life-saving medical therapy that should be administered as quickly as possible to try to restore blood flow to the heart. After a heart attack, cardiac rehabilitation is an essential part of the treatment. The long-term therapies for those who have suffered a heart attack are the same as for those with coronary artery disease, as we discussed earlier in this chapter.

Lifestyle Changes

♥ Cardiac rehabilitation: Anyone recovering from a heart attack should complete cardiac rehabilitation. Not only does cardiac rehab provide a monitored setting in which you can exercise and regain your strength, it also offers emotional support and education. Cardiac rehabilitation will reduce your risk for a future heart attack, in addition to reducing your risk of dying.

Medications

♥ Aspirin: This medication should be given immediately when a heart attack is suspected, as it improves the chances of survival.

♥ Beta blockers: This type of medication should be taken immediately when a heart attack is occurring to slow the heart rate and the workload of the heart. Beta blockers have been shown to improve survival if given early and prevent subsequent heart attacks from occurring.

♥ ACE inhibitors: These medications should be started soon after a heart attack, as they have been proven to reduce the damage to the heart and improve survival after a heart attack. Their long-term use reduces the risk of future heart attacks and improves the chances of survival should one occur.

♥ Statins: These medications, particularly high-dose statins, should be started as soon as possible after a heart attack as they can improve the chances of survival.

♥ Nitrates: While nitrates do not improve the chances of survival, they can relieve symptoms of angina.

♥ Thrombolytics: In the ideal situation, a person suffering a heart attack would have a *cardiac catheterization*, where the heart arteries are examined and any blocked artery is opened using angioplasty and kept open with a stent. However, hospitals that are unable to perform this procedure will use thrombolytics, which are clot-busting agents, to open the blocked artery and restore blood flow to the heart. They should be given within three hours of a heart attack. The earlier the medication is taken, the greater the chance of surviving the heart attack.

♥ Anti-platelet agents: In addition to aspirin, anti-platelet agents such as clopidogrel (Plavix) are often given after a heart attack with or without a coronary artery stent, as this has been proven to improve the chance of survival. In addition, when a heart attack is diagnosed, medications called platelet glycoprotein IIb/IIIa receptor blockers can be started to reduce the risk of new blood clots forming. Intravenous heparin or an injection of low-molecular-weight heparin will be administered in the emergency room if a heart attack is suspected. (See Chapter 5 for more information on all of these medications.)

♥ Painkillers: If the chest pain associated with a heart attack is too great, painkillers such as morphine may be used.

♥ Omega-3 fatty acids: After a heart attack, taking omega-3 fatty acids improves survival and reduces the risk of sudden cardiac death, as discussed in the previous section on coronary artery disease. It is useful to start this medication after a heart attack to lower the risk of either of these occurring.

Generally, women wait longer than men to go to an emergency room when having a heart attack. And physicians are slower to recognize the presence of heart attacks in women because "characteristic" patterns of chest pain and ECG changes are less frequently present. Women, in general, as well as people with diabetes and older adults, may not have the classic symptom of chest pain that is usually associated with a heart attack. They are more likely to suffer from shortness of breath, nausea, back pain, and/or jaw pain.

Treatment Goals

For a person who is having a heart attack, the goals of treatment are to stabilize the patient, remove the blood clot that is causing the heart attack, minimize the damage to the heart, relieve the person's symptoms, and improve her chances of surviving the heart attack. Additional goals are also to work toward improving the person's chances for long-term survival and reducing her risks of future cardiac events.

> After a heart attack, women are less likely than men to receive beta blockers, ACE inhibitors, and aspirin — therapies proven to improve survival. This contributes to a higher rate of complications and a higher death rate after a heart attack in women overall.

Heart Failure

Definition: Inability of the heart to pump blood to meet the demands of the body.

Therapeutic Options

The goal of therapy for a person with heart failure is to stabilize or improve the heart function. In addition, therapy also aims to treat any symptoms that may be present.

Lifestyle Changes

- ♥ Diet: Eat a heart-healthy diet that is low in salt (less than 2 grams per day); avoid drinking alcohol; and avoid caffeine intake since this can increase your heart rate and thereby increase the demands on your heart.
- ♥ Exercise: Be sure to exercise daily to improve the symptoms of heart failure. It prevents deconditioning and may improve your heart function over time.
- ♥ Smoking: If you smoke, stop. Smoking raises your heart rate, increasing the demands on an already poorly functioning heart. Smoking will raise blood pressure and also can damage the arteries of the heart, causing further damage to the heart and its function.
- ♥ Fluid intake: Know that when you have heart failure, the body's tendency is to retain fluid. By measuring your weight daily and

monitoring your fluid intake, you can better know how much liquid you should be taking in. This will also help your medical management, by allowing your doctor to determine how much of a diuretic you may need to prevent your symptoms from worsening.

♥ Blood pressure, cholesterol, and diabetes control: Ensure all of these conditions are controlled and monitored as part of reducing your risk of a stroke in the future. Discuss with your doctor what means of control are right for you.

♥ Annual flu vaccine and one-time pneumococcal vaccine: Consider getting these vaccines. They are beneficial for those with heart failure, as any severe illness can stress the heart further.

Medications

♥ ACE inhibitors: These drugs are proven to improve heart function and increase the chances of long-term survival in those with heart failure.

♥ Angiotensin II receptor blockers (ARBs): These drugs work like ACE inhibitors to improve heart function in the case of heart failure and are used when ACE inhibitors are not tolerated.

♥ Beta blockers: These drugs improve the chances of survival for a person suffering heart failure. Beta blockers shown to improve outcomes include carvedilol (Coreg), metoprolol succinate (Toprol XL), and bisoprolol (Zebeta, Concor).

♥ Hydralazine plus nitrates: This combination does improve the chances of survival but appears less powerful than ACE inhibitors. Often it is given to those who cannot take ACE inhibitors or ABRs, or it is used in combination with these drugs. Studies have shown that hydralazine plus nitrates is particularly useful in people of African descent who have heart failure.

♥ Diuretics: These drugs provide relief of symptoms of heart failure (shortness of breath, weight gain, ankle or leg swelling, etc.) by removing fluid from the body through the kidneys, but do not affect survival. Lasix (furosemide) is the most common diuretic.

♥ Aldosterone inhibitors: These drugs are proven to reduce the need for hospitalization and improve the chances of survival for those with symptoms of heart failure.

♥ Digoxin: This medication provides relief of the symptoms of heart failure but does not affect a person's chances of survival.

♥ Omega-3 fatty acids: There is increasing evidence that omega-3 fatty acids (fish oil is a good source) may be beneficial for people with heart failure. A landmark study in 2008 showed a reduction in hospitalization and improved survival in patients with heart failure who took 1 gram of omega-3 fatty acid daily.[5]

♥ Acute treatment (intravenous medications): If a person is hospitalized with heart failure that is worsening and she is not responding to standard therapies, intravenous drugs such as dobutamine, nitroglycerine, nitroprusside, milrinone, or nesiritide may be used to try to improve the heart's pumping function and try to get blood flowing to the entire body.

Devices

♥ Implantable cardioverter defibrillator (ICD): An ICD is a defibrillator that is implanted under the skin and has wires placed into the heart that work to shock the heart back into a normal heart rhythm if a dangerous, life-threatening arrhythmia occurs or if the heart stops beating. Not everyone with heart failure needs an ICD, but an ICD may be recommended when the *ejection fraction* of the heart (the fraction of blood that is squeezed forward to the arteries to bring blood to the body — the *contraction*) is quite low (less than 35%) or when there has been an episode of sudden cardiac death (also called cardiac arrest; when the heart fails to pump blood). In these cases, an ICD can be a live-saving device, because the risk of a repeat cardiac arrest is high.

♥ Cardiac resynchronization therapy (CRT): When heart failure is due to an abnormality in the heart's electrical conducting system, a CRT can be implanted under the skin with wires placed in the heart to correct the conduction so that both ventricles beat together. This is a specialized pacemaker that has been proven to improve symptoms, improve the function of the heart, and improve the chances of survival in those with heart failure.

♥ Left ventricular assist device (LVAD): This pumping device is surgically implanted when the left ventricle is failing to keep up with the demands of the body and medications are not working. It is amazing technology that has grown quickly and is keeping people alive and out of the hospital. Some people with this device get a heart transplant at a later time, but many will not. The device can extend a person's life and allow them to go home, where in the past they had to be hospitalized or would die. (Interesting fact: The former vice-president Dick Cheney got this device implanted in the summer of 2010.)

Treatment Goals
Treatment for heart failure is aimed at improving the patient's symptoms, improving heart function, and improving survival. Heart failure from any cause can increase the risk of sudden cardiac death, arrhythmias, and worsening heart function. All these issues are addressed when deciding which medications a heart failure patient would benefit from.

Heart Arrhythmias
Definition: Abnormal heart rates or rhythms.

Therapeutic Options
Heart arrhythmias are complex, ranging from benign and requiring no treatment to arrhythmias that can be deadly. Thus, the treatments vary for the particular condition.

Lifestyle Changes
♥ Caffeine: Reduce your intake of caffeine from any source, be it coffee, black or green tea, chocolate, and even some medications, because caffeine can trigger skipped heartbeats and certain arrhythmias. Cutting caffeine from your diet may resolve the issue.

♥ Stimulants: Avoid taking any stimulants, which cause your heart to beat faster and can provoke serious arrhythmias. Examples of such drugs are pseudoephedrine, amphetamine, and dextroamphetamine. Avoid certain cold and nasal medications that can have stimulants in them; read the label and avoid anything that contains *pseudoephedrine*. Cocaine and amphetamines also can be very dangerous to the heart.

♥ Smoking: Know that nicotine, found in cigarettes, is a stimulant and can provoke heart rhythm problems.

♥ Stress: Remember that this common affliction may be a trigger for your symptoms. If it is, work to reduce your stress (see Chapter 10).

♥ Alcohol: Avoid drinking excessive amounts (more than four drinks for a woman) of alcohol in one sitting (*binge drinking*), which can bring on certain types of arrhythmias.

♥ Thyroid disorder control: If you have a known thyroid disorder, make sure your thyroid levels are normal. If you don't have a known thyroid issue, ask your doctor to have your thyroid levels checked (by blood work), as thyroid hormone levels affect metabolism, and abnormalities in metabolism can result in heart rhythm abnormalities.

♥ Vagal maneuvers: These simple but effective actions — holding your breath, bearing down or straining, coughing — can slow the heart rate down and help resolve certain arrhythmias.

Medications

A variety of medications may be used to treat heart arrhythmias, depending on the diagnosis of the heart rhythm disturbance and its underlying cause. The medications often work to slow down the heart or suppress the abnormal rhythm from taking over from the normal rhythm. Some arrhythmias (such as atrial fibrillation) increase the risk of a stroke; an anticoagulant may be required to reduce this risk.

♥ Beta blockers or calcium channel blockers: The aim of these drugs is to slow the heart rate. Less commonly, a medication called digoxin may be used to slow the heart rate.

♥ Anti-arrhythmics: These drugs work to suppress or prevent the arrhythmia by either slowing the electrical conduction through the heart or suppressing the electrical signal that triggers the arrhythmia.

♥ Anti-coagulants: Atrial fibrillation is a particular type of arrhythmia that increases a person's risk of a stroke. Depending on an individual's risk, either of two anti-coagulants may be recommended: aspirin for those considered at lower risk for a stroke and warfarin for those considered at higher risk.

♥ Medications to control cardiac risk factors: Controlling hypertension, high cholesterol, and any other risk factors is important, because having an arrhythmia places you at a higher risk of having a heart attack or stroke. Discuss with your doctor what medications might help you control your cardiac risk factors.

Devices

♥ Pacemaker: This device is implanted under the skin in the chest area and it has wires that are attached to the heart. It is battery powered and will work to increase the heart rate when it senses the heart rate is too slow. A pacemaker is used when the heart rate is persistently low and the person has symptoms (lightheadedness, dizziness, passing out, shortness of breath, chest pain, weakness, or fatigue) because inadequate amounts of blood are being pumped to meet what the body and its organs need. It can also be used when the top chambers of the heart (the atria) are not communicating with the lower chambers (the ventricles), in cases of heart block.

♥ Implantable cardioverter defibrillator (ICD): This device is similar to a pacemaker and has pacemaker capabilities, but it is implanted when there is a high risk of a dangerous, life-threatening arrhythmia. The ICD will sense this risk and shock the heart to try to restore a normal rhythm.

Treatment Goals

The goal of any treatment of an arrhythmia is not only to reduce your symptoms but also reduce the risks associated with the arrhythmia. In addition, if medications are needed to treat the arrhythmia, their benefits must outweigh their risks. Many anti-arrhythmic medications have serious side effects; your doctor must monitor your condition whether you take these medications for the short term or if you remain on them for some time. If lifestyle changes and drugs are ineffective at treating the heart rhythm disturbance or if you cannot tolerate the medication, you may need an electrophysiology (EP) study (see Chapter 4). Such procedures, when successful, can prevent the long-term use of medication.

Ischemic Stroke

Definition: The result of a blood clot that blocks an artery leading to an area of the brain; when this occurs, the brain tissue can start dying.

Therapeutic Options

The acute treatment for ischemic stroke is aimed to restore blood flow to the brain and reduce the amount of permanent damage that is sustained. Ultimately, time is of the essence, because like the heart, the brain requires blood flow for oxygen and other nutrients. Long-term therapy aims to reduce the risk of a future stroke and reduce the impact of any disabilities caused by the initial stroke.

Lifestyle Changes

♥ Diet: Eat heart-healthy foods (include lots of vegetables, fruit, whole grains, and fiber, and eat omega-3–rich fish twice a week). Reduce the amount of LDL (bad) cholesterol in your diet.

♥ Exercise: Get regular daily exercise to help reduce your risk of having a stroke or subsequent stroke if you've already had one. Even if you have physical limitations after a stroke, it is important to get help to remain physically active.

♥ Smoking: Remember that smoking is a risk factor for stroke. For those who have had an initial stroke, not quitting smoking can result in another stroke.

♥ Birth control: Know that women who have had a stroke while on the birth control pill must not take the pill or any other hormones, whether oral or transdermal.

♥ Hormone replacement therapy: Women who have had a stroke or TIA must avoid taking hormone replacement therapy.

♥ Blood pressure, cholesterol, and diabetes control: Be sure that your risk factors, all of which are part of reducing your risk of stroke, are controlled. Discuss with your doctor what means of control are right for you.

Medications

♥ Thrombolytics: In cases when a stroke has been caught early, the thrombolytic tPA is used as part of the acute treatment. It must be administered within three hours from when the stroke began. Thrombolytics are essentially "clot-busters" that will break down the clot and restore the blood flow to the brain. Unfortunately, only a small percentage (3 to 5%) of persons who have a stroke get treated with this medication because few people make it to the hospital in time.

♥ Anti-platelet agents: Aspirin is often taken after a stroke. Depending on the source of the blood clot, warfarin may be used. Aspirin is useful in women for stroke prevention and is recommended for women age 65 and older.

Treatment Goals

Once a stroke has occurred, the focus is on preventing another stroke. All risk factors must be well controlled to reduce the risk of a subsequent stroke. Although strokes occur more frequently in men than women, women are more likely to die from a stroke. In addition, treatment to regain independence and physical activity are part of the treatment regimen.

Peripheral Arterial Disease (PAD)

Definition: Blockage of the arteries in the extremities of the body, especially in the legs.

Therapeutic Options

A diagnosis of PAD is usually based on the symptom of leg pain when walking (*intermittent claudication*). This symptom is usually reproducible: when walking a certain distance, someone with PAD will have to stop to get relief from the pain. So treatment must focus on relieving pain, as well as on treating the disease.

Lifestyle Changes

♥ Smoking: Know that quitting smoking is the most important change you can make after receiving a diagnosis of PAD. Smokers have four times greater the risk of PAD than nonsmokers. Quitting smoking will slow the progression of PAD and reduce the risks to your heart.

♥ Diet: Eat a heart-healthy diet (rich in fruits and vegetables, whole grains, fiber, lean meats, and omega-3–rich fish twice a week) that is low in saturated fats, trans fats, and dietary cholesterol. (See Chapter 8 for more about eating for heart health.)

♥ Exercise: Be aware that exercise is the most effective treatment for PAD. It can reduce your symptoms of pain and improve blood flow in the arteries in the legs. Exercise needs to be built up slowly and guided by a healthcare professional, as walking causes pain in PAD sufferers.

Medications

♥ Anti-platelets: Since PAD is essentially excessive plaque formation (*atherosclerosis*) of the leg arteries, some anti-platelet agent should be used to thin the blood, either aspirin or clopidogrel (Plavix) or both.

♥ Medication to improve claudication: Medications that work to improve blood circulation in the legs may be used to relieve leg pain while walking (*claudication*). Examples are pentoxifylline (Trental) and cilostazol (Pletal).

♥ Medication to treat and control of high blood pressure, high cholesterol, and diabetes: Controlling these conditions plays a part of reducing your risk of a stroke in the future. Discuss with your doctor what means of control are right for you.

Treatment Goals

In those with PAD, the goals of treatment are to reduce the symptoms (mainly the pain) and to slow or reverse the progression of the disease.

Heart Risk Factors
High Blood Pressure (Hypertension)

Definition: Blood pressure in the arteries that is persistently higher than normal, resulting in artery damage and can cause a heart attack or stroke.

Therapeutic Options

Treatment of high blood pressure will lower your risk of a heart attack and stroke and prevent damage to your kidneys and your heart, which lowers the risk of developing heart failure. The effects of lifestyle changes in particular cannot be overstated. If you made all the changes we suggest here, you would lower your blood pressure beyond what any one medication could do, lowering your systolic blood pressure by 21 to 55 mmHg (millimeters of mercury, which is how blood pressure is measured), significantly lowering your risk of a stroke or heart attack with lifestyle changes alone.

Lifestyle Changes

♥ Low-salt/DASH diet: Follow a low-salt (*low-sodium*) diet to dramatically lower your blood pressure. In particular, adhering to the Dietary Approaches to Stop Hypertension (DASH) diet, which includes both dietary changes and a low-salt regimen (3 grams or less of salt per day), is proven to reduce blood pressure in people with normal blood pressure and is even more effective in lowering blood pressure in people with hypertension. The DASH diet alone has been shown to decrease systolic blood pressure by 6 mmHg and the diastolic blood pressure by 3 mmHg. If an even lower-salt diet (less than 1.5 grams daily) is adhered to in conjunction with the DASH diet, systolic blood pressure can drop by an additional 4 mmHg. This is equivalent to the usual response of any hypertension-lowering medication. A low-salt diet (less than 1.5 grams daily) is recommended as the first line of treatment for hypertension.

♥ Exercise: Get regular physical activity for 30 minutes a day, every day, and you will see systolic blood pressure drop by 4 to 9 mmHg. If you exercise in addition to following the DASH diet, blood pressure can drop by 16/10 mmHg.

♥ Weight loss: If you have an elevated body mass index (see Chapter 2), lose weight to improve your blood pressure (never mind your waistline!). For every 22 pounds (10 kilograms) of weight loss, the average reduction in systolic blood pressure is between 5 and 20 mmHg.

♥ Smoking: Quit smoking to improve blood pressure. Although smoking itself does not cause high blood pressure, your blood pressure is temporarily raised each time you smoke.

♥ Alcohol: Limit the amount of alcohol you drink to less than one alcoholic drink per day. One drink is considered to be 5 ounces (142 ml) of wine, 12 ounces (340 ml) of regular beer, or 1 1/2 ounces (45 ml) of hard liquor. Reducing your alcohol consumption may reduce your systolic blood pressure by 2 to 4 mmHg.

Medications

♥ Diuretics: These are some of the oldest and simplest drugs that are usually well tolerated. They are the recommended first line of therapy for high blood pressure, and are discussed in detail in Chapter 5 (as are the other drugs listed below).

♥ Beta blockers

♥ Calcium channel blockers

♥ Aldosterone inhibitors

♥ Angiotensin inhibitors (ACE inhibitors)

♥ Angiotensin II receptor blockers (ARBs)

♥ Renin inhibitors

♥ Alpha blockers

♥ Alpha agonists

♥ Combination therapy: There are many combination drugs available, combining two classes of drug, for ease of use. The fact is that most people need more than one medication to control their blood pressure, so these combinations simply make life easier. However, they are often more expensive than single-purpose medications.

Treatment Goals

Ultimately, the goal of any treatment (lifestyle changes with or without medications) is to get your blood pressure to the target number to lower your risk of cardiovascular disease. The targets are set based on whether your issues are complicated or not. (By complicated, we mean if you already have heart disease or have had a stroke, or known organ damage from long-standing high blood pressure.) Diabetics are at increased risk of organ damage and heart disease, so blood pressure control is paramount in diabetics and their blood pressure goals are tighter.

Blood Pressure Targets Based on Risk

	Target blood pressure (systolic/diastolic)
Uncomplicated high blood pressure (isolated high blood pressure with no organ damage)	<140/90 mmHg
Complicated high blood pressure (high blood pressure with cardiovascular disease, diabetes, or other organ damage, such as kidney damage)	<130/80 mmHg

High Cholesterol (Hyperlipidemia)
Definition: Abnormally elevated levels of cholesterol in the blood.

Therapeutic Options
Abnormal cholesterol levels, particularly an elevation in LDL cholesterol, result in excessive plaque formation (*atherosclerosis*) in the arteries leading to the heart and brain. Knowing and controlling your cholesterol through lifestyle changes — the first line of treatment — and possibly medication are the keys to reducing your risk of a heart attack and stroke.

Lifestyle Changes
♥ Diet: See if changing your diet can prevent you from needing medications to treat high cholesterol. This is *always* the first step to lowering cholesterol. Eating a high-fiber diet rich in vegetables, fruits, whole grains, and lean meats, and eating omega-3–rich fish twice a week can improve your cholesterol. It is also important to watch your consumption of fat, particularly saturated fats and trans fats, and dietary cholesterol.
♥ Exercise: Get regular exercise — at least 30 minutes a day — to have profound effects on blood cholesterol levels by raising the HDL (good) cholesterol and lowering LDL (bad) cholesterol and triglycerides.
♥ Smoking: Quit smoking to raise your HDL cholesterol levels.

Medications

There are a number of medications that can be used to improve your cholesterol, depending on where the problem lies. The table below summarizes the available drugs' effects on cholesterol and their possible side effects. For each drug, we give the chemical name followed by the brand name in parentheses. The arrows indicate whether there is an increasing (↑), lowering (↓), or no significant change (↔) effect on the cholesterol. Double arrows reflect a more profound effect on lowering or raising the specific cholesterol levels.

Benefits and Side Effects of Cholesterol-Lowering Drugs

Drug class	Drug names	Benefits	Possible side effects
Statins	atorvastatin (Lipitor) fluvastatin (Lescol) lovastatin (Mevacor) pravastatin (Pravacol) rosuvastatin (Crestor) simvastatin (Zocor)	↓↓ LDL ↑ HDL ↓ triglycerides	Muscle aches/ pain ↑ liver enzymes
Cholesterol absorption inhibitors	**Resins (bile acid-binding)** cholestyramine (Questran, Questran Light, Prevalite, Locholest, Locholest Light) colestipol (Colestid) colesevelam (Welchol)	↓ LDL ↑ HDL ↔ triglycerides	Diarrhea Flatulence Constipation
	Selective inhibitor ezetimibe (Zetia in the United States; Ezetrol in Canada)	↓ LDL ↑ /↔ HDL ↔ triglycerides	Stomach upset Muscle aches/ pain ↑ Liver enzymes
Nicotinic acid*	niacin* (Niacin, Niaspan)	↓ LDL ↑↑ HDL ↓↓ triglycerides	Flushing ↑ liver enzymes Gout (may worsen diabetes)
Fibrinic acids	clofibrate (Atromid-S) fenofibrate (Tricor) fenofibric acid (Trilipix) gemfibrozil (Lopid)	↓ LDL ↑ HDL ↓↓ triglycerides	Muscle aches/ pain Gallstones Dyspepsia

continued on next page

| Omega-3 fatty acids docosahexaenoic acid (DHA) eicosapentaenoic acid (EPA) | omega-3 ester (Lovaza) | ↑ LDL ↑ HDL ↓↓ triglycerides | Flu-like symptoms Belching Stomach upset Rash Change in taste |

*Niacin is available both as a prescription and as an off-the-shelf dietary supplement. We do not recommend using the dietary supplement as a substitute for prescription niacin when trying to lower cholesterol. The supplement is not regulated in the same way as is the prescription form and contains variable amounts of active niacin (from as little as none to more than the label claims). "No-flush" niacin has inactivated the ingredient needed to lower your cholesterol.

Statins tend to be the medication of choice in treating high cholesterol, because effectiveness and safety is strongest with this class of drug. They have been shown to reduce the risk of a heart attack and other major cardiovascular issues for those with heart disease (secondary prevention) and those who do not have heart disease (primary prevention). Studies of this drug included women and have shown that statins are very effective medications for women.

Treatment Goals

Treatment goals for LDL cholesterol are based on risk factors and risk assessment. To calculate your 10-year risk of developing heart disease, see Chapter 3. If your treatment goals are not achieved through lifestyle changes, you will need medications and your fasting cholesterol (and liver tests to assess for drug side effects) will need to be followed to assess your response to any therapy (usually within six to eight weeks to see the effect of medication). Once treatment goals are achieved, cholesterol (and the liver) will be checked every six months or more frequently if there is a change in your diet, medication tolerance or compliance, or weight.

LDL Goals and Treatment Based on Risk Profile[6]

Risk category	LDL goal	LDL level at which to initiate lifestyle changes (mg/dL)*	LDL level at which to initiate drug therapy (mg/dL)
Heart disease or high risk (10-year risk >20%)	<100 mg/dL (<2.6 mmol/L**) [or in some cases, <70 mg/dL (<1.8 mmol/L) applies]	>100 mg/dL (>2.6 mmol/L)	>130 mg/dL (>3.4 mmol/L)

>2 risk factors (10- year risk <20%)	<130 mg/dL (<3.4 mmol/L)	>130 mg/dL (>3.4 mmol/L)	10-year risk 10–20% >130 mg/dL (>3.4 mmol/L)
			10-year risk <10% >160 mg/dL (>4.1 mmol/L)
0–1 risk factor	<160 mg/dL (<4.1 mmol/L)	>160 mg/dL (>4.1 mmol/L)	>190 mg/dL (>4.9 mmol/L)

*milligrams/deciliter (the measure used in the United States)
**millimoles/liter (the metric measure used in Canada and Europe)

For HDL, the optimal level for women is above 50 mg/dL (>1.3mmol/L); lower levels have been associated with a higher risk of heart disease. Reducing trans fats, quitting smoking, and exercise can raise HDL levels, as can some of the medications listed above.

For those with highly elevated levels of triglycerides, defined as >500 mg/dL (>5.7 mmol/L), the primary goal of treatment is to lower those levels. LDL cholesterol, however, cannot be accurately measured when the blood is so thick and full of triglycerides; they prevent the lab from distinguishing the LDL particles. But LDL is not important at this time because the primary focus of treatment is to reduce the triglycerides. Lifestyle changes and medications are used to get triglyceride levels controlled. Particular lifestyle changes, especially changes in diet, are meant to reduce your intake not only of saturated fat but also simple carbohydrates, which can raise triglycerides significantly. Poorly controlled diabetes is often associated with an elevated triglyceride level and low level of HDL cholesterol. Medications that are effective at lowering triglycerides are niacin, fibrates, statins, and omega-3 fatty acids.

Diabetes
Definition: The inability of the body to regulate levels of glucose, resulting in elevated blood glucose levels. This occurs as a result of resistance to or insufficient amounts of the hormone insulin.

Therapeutic Options
Sixty-five percent of diabetics die from heart disease and stroke. So it's clear that avoiding diabetes altogether is preferable. But if you have diabetes, making sure it is well controlled can reduce your risk of a heart

attack or stroke. A combination of lifestyle changes and medication can achieve this. Controlling or avoiding diabetes is particularly important in women, since a woman with diabetes is at much greater risk of cardiovascular disease than a man with diabetes.

Lifestyle Changes
♥ Weight control: Work to attain and maintain a healthy weight to help prevent the onset of diabetes or improve diabetes control if you already have the disease.
♥ Diet: Eat healthy foods (include lots of vegetables and complex fiber in your diet, eat omega-3–rich fish twice a week) and reduce your sugar and simple carbohydrate intake. Also, reduce your cholesterol and alcohol intake. You may want to consider working with a dietitian to help you get better control over your diabetes.
♥ Exercise: Regular daily exercise can improve your body's blood sugar control and delay the progression of diabetes.

Medications
♥ Work with your physician to find the optimal medications for you to treat and keep your diabetes well controlled. There are a variety of medications that can be used. You may also consider working with a diabetes educator to help you get better control of your diabetes. If you need additional help, you may be advised to see a doctor who specializes in diabetes (*endocrinologist*).
♥ If you have diabetes, you are at high risk for heart disease and should be treated like anyone with heart disease. This means you need the standard of care medication recommended for anyone with coronary artery disease: a daily aspirin, an ACE inhibitor, and a statin targeting your LDL cholesterol to get it under 100 mg/dL (and optimally under 70 mg/dL).

Treatment Goals
Your *hemoglobin A1c* reading (HbA1c — see Chapter 4) tells you the average blood sugar in your system over the past three months. The target HbA1c should be less than 7% for all diabetics.

The Heart of the Matter

Keep taking the medicine

Patient: It's been one month since my last visit and I still feel miserable.

Doctor: Did you follow the instructions on the medicine I gave you?

Patient: I sure did—the bottle said, "Keep tightly closed."

— Anonymous

Our words of advice are to take your medication. Do not stop medications once you have met your treatment goals unless advised to do so by your doctor. In most cases, stopping the medication will reverse the effect of the drug that has gotten you to that goal, and sometimes stopping a medication can be very dangerous. If your medication is causing unwanted side effects, let your pharmacist and doctor know. Sometimes these side effects can be minimized; other times the adverse effects will eventually diminish. If you can't tolerate the drug, speak to your doctor and pharmacist so that you can work toward finding the right medication for you. Until doctors have a genetic map of their patients' drug tolerances (yes, it is coming one day!), finding the drug that works best for you is sometimes a matter of trial and error. And the good news is that with modern medicine, we have many choices of drugs. We have patients for whom it took up to two years to find the best medication regime to control their blood pressure or cholesterol, but we finally found it. In most cases, it won't take that long, but if it does, remember: perseverance (and a little patience) *will* pay off.

Chapter 7

Nature's Pharmacy

In all things of Nature, there is something of the marvelous.
— Aristotle

Medicine has evolved significantly in the past few centuries, from the discovery and use of plants for healing to the development and boom of patented pharmaceuticals. The use of plants for healing is an ancient practice that dates back over 60,000 years. Berries, roots, seeds, flowers, and other parts of plants provided our ancestors with a wide range of medicines. As science and medical knowledge expanded, therapeutic compounds were identified from plants, extracted, and made into drugs. Still today, plants are the primary medicines used in many countries around the world — China, Japan, and India, as well as throughout Africa — and in North America there is a renewed interest in using plants and other naturally derived products.

Herbal remedies, vitamins, fatty acids, probiotics, and other supplements are classified today as "dietary supplements" (in the United States) or "natural health products" (in Canada).

Consumer sales of dietary supplements in the United States alone were estimated at $25.2 billion in 2008.[1] Surveys reveal that approximately 50 to 70% of North Americans regularly take dietary supplements.[2] The most common reasons why people take these supplements are to stay healthy and to prevent or treat certain health problems.

Mounting clinical research is demonstrating that certain supplements can play an important role in promoting health and preventing disease. Every day, research sheds more light on the health benefits of various vitamins, plants, and food-based compounds, as well as the safety and efficacy of these products.

Plants as medicine

Hundreds of the drugs in use today are derived directly from plants or contain synthesized materials from agents originally derived from plants. For example, the widely used drug for congestive heart failure digoxin is derived from Digitalis purpurea, *commonly known as purple foxglove. Quinidine, a drug used for cardiac arrhythmia (irregular heart rhythm), is derived from the quinine tree,* Cinchone ledgeriana.

Many people today are looking for healing methods beyond drug therapy or for approaches that can be used in conjunction with conventional medicine. There is no debate that most people with chronic diseases can be greatly helped by lifestyle approaches, such as healthy eating, stress management, exercise, and adequate sleep. In addition to lifestyle, many people are exploring the benefits of acupuncture, chiropractic treatments, and other natural healing methods. Nutritional supplements are also recognized as having a valuable role in supporting health. Supplements, when taken appropriately, can complement lifestyle approaches, make up for deficiencies or gaps in the diet, and help protect against chronic diseases, such as heart disease.

Conventional healthcare practitioners are also embracing the role that nutritional supplements can play in promoting health and preventing disease and they are making recommendations for their patients. Once seen as "alternative," many of these products are now considered part of the mainstream approach to health, and many practitioners integrate conventional and natural medicine into treating patients.

The art of healing comes from nature and not from the physician. Therefore, the physician must start from nature with an open mind.
— Paracelsus

The shelves of pharmacies and health food stores are lined with countless nutritional supplements. As a consumer, it can be daunting to figure out which products to take and how to take them properly. Are supplements regulated? Are these products backed by clinical research? Are there any side effects or precautions? How do you choose one product over another? In this chapter we answer these questions, provide information on specific supplements that may be beneficial for heart health and those that should be avoided, and we provide tips on safe supplementing.

Are Dietary Supplements Regulated?

In 1994, the U.S. Congress enacted the Dietary Supplements Health and Education Act (DSHEA). Before the passage of the DSHEA, dietary supplements were considered foods and were subject to the same regulatory requirements as foods. The new law established separate guidelines for the safety and regulation of dietary supplements. According to the DSHEA, a dietary supplement is "a product that is intended to supplement the diet and bears or contains one or more of the following dietary ingredients: a vitamin, a mineral, an herb or other botanical, an amino acid, a dietary substance for use by man to supplement the diet by increasing the total daily intake, or a concentrate, metabolite, constituent, or extract."[3]

The DSHEA granted the Food and Drug Administration (FDA) oversight responsibility, and requires ingredient and nutrition labeling for all dietary supplements. The law also set up rules governing safety, advertising, and label claim issues. Under the DSHEA, a manufacturer is responsible for determining that the dietary supplements it manufactures or distributes are safe and that any representations or claims made about them are substantiated by adequate evidence to show that they are not false or misleading. This means that dietary supplements do not need approval from the FDA before they are marketed. Except in the case of a new dietary ingredient, where the law requires a pre-market review for safety data and other information, a manufacturer does not have to provide the FDA with the evidence it relies on to substantiate safety or effectiveness before or after it markets its products.

In Canada, the government established the Natural Health Products Directorate (NHPD) as the regulating authority for natural health products for sale in Canada. Its role is to ensure that Canadians have ready access to natural health products that are safe, effective, and of high quality. The NHPD establishes regulations on product licensing, manufacturing practices, adverse reaction reporting, clinical trials, labeling, and provisions for health claims. Under the Natural Health Products Regulations, which came into effect January 1, 2004, natural health products (NHPs) are defined as vitamins and minerals, herbal remedies, homeopathic medicines, traditional medicines such as traditional Chinese medicines, probiotics, and other products like amino acids and essential fatty acids. NHPs must be as safe as over-the-counter products and not require a prescription to be sold.[4]

Why Take Supplements?

You may have heard people say, "If you eat a healthy diet, you don't need to take supplements." If you eat a whole-foods diet, with plenty of nutrient-dense, organic fruits and vegetables, whole grains, lean protein, and healthy fats every day, it may be possible to get what your body needs from diet alone. However, the reality is that not many people eat this way on a regular basis. With our busy lifestyles, fast foods and processed foods are prevalent in our diet, and these foods are typically devoid of nutrients. Furthermore, our bodies can become depleted of nutrients in numerous ways — for example, through stress, environmental toxins (pesticides), and even prescription medication use.

Nutritional supplements not only help make up for dietary deficiencies and nutrient depletion but also support health and help prevent chronic disease. It is important to keep in mind, though, that supplements are intended to *complement*, not *replace*, a healthy lifestyle: You can't eat poorly and live unhealthily and expect a supplement to compensate for those choices.

A review of 41 studies comparing 35 vitamin and mineral levels of organic and conventional produce revealed that organic produce ranked higher in most nutrients measured. The top three nutritional differences were magnesium, vitamin C, and iron (organics had 29, 27, and 21% more, respectively).[5]

Creating Your Supplement Program

With so many supplements available, if you took everything that sounds beneficial, you would end up popping pills all day long. Take into account your diet, lifestyle, and health needs when determining what supplements to take. A few supplements can be considered foundation supplements. These include multivitamins and minerals, green food supplements, and omega-3 fatty acids, all of which offer a broad range of health benefits.

Multivitamins and Minerals

Multivitamins provide a range of vitamins, minerals, and other nutritional elements that are considered beneficial for health. Taking a daily multivitamin helps ensure that your body gets all the essential nutrients it needs to function optimally. Aside from a poor diet, there are many factors that increase your need for vitamins and minerals, such as smoking, use of prescription medication, intense exercise, stress, and certain medical conditions, for example, osteoporosis, alcoholism, and malabsorption diseases (such as celiac and Crohn's diseases). Even if you eat a healthy diet, you could still be lacking in certain nutrients. And those on a strict vegetarian diet may have difficulty getting enough essential nutrients through food alone.

There are multivitamin formulas that are designed specifically for children, pregnant women, active adults, and seniors. Because nutritional needs vary with age, gender, and lifestyle, it is important to look for a multivitamin designed for your particular needs. For example:

♥ Women of child-bearing age may need extra iron, especially if they have heavy menstrual cycles.

♥ Women who are planning to become pregnant or are pregnant or lactating should take a prenatal multivitamin, which contains higher amounts of nutrients needed to support the growing baby and meet the increased demands of breast-feeding.

♥ Athletes may require extra antioxidants to compensate for free radicals generated during intense activity.

♥ Seniors require extra calcium and vitamin D to protect their bones, and to possibly reduce their risk of heart disease, particularly if they are vitamin D deficient. Vitamin B12 can be deficient in older individuals depending on diet, medical conditions, and prescription drug use. Most seniors should not take multivitamins containing iron unless advised by their doctor.

Green Foods
Most people find it difficult to consume the recommended servings of fruits and vegetables per day. To complement your diet, you may want to consider taking a green foods supplement. Green foods such as chlorella, spirulina, barley grass, and wheat grass provide vital nutrients, including antioxidants and minerals, along with fiber and plant compounds, which can help boost energy levels, support detoxification, and enhance well-being. There are many green food supplements on the market, which vary in composition. Some brands to consider are Kyo-Greens and greens+. You can add the greens to your morning protein shake or simply mix with juice or water.

Omega-3 Fatty Acids
There are different types of dietary fats (see Chapter 8). Some are good for health, others are detrimental. Saturated fats and trans fats are the bad fats that we need to minimize in our diet. Unsaturated fatty acids, namely monounsaturated and polyunsaturated fatty acids, are beneficial fats. The two main classes of polyunsaturated are *omega-3* (alpha-linolenic) and *omega-6* (linoleic) *fatty acids*. These fats are known as *essential fatty acids* (EFAs) because they are essential for our health. The body converts alpha-linolenic acid (ALA) into the longer chain fatty acids eicosapentaenoic acid (EPA) and docosahexaenoic acid (DHA). Our bodies need EFAs for growth and development of the brain, nervous system, adrenal glands, sex organs, and eyes. EFAs maintain the health of cell membranes, produce hormones and brain chemicals, and regulate various cell processes. The body cannot make its own EFAs, so we must obtain them through diet or supplementation.

Most people get adequate omega-6s, as they are found abundantly in vegetable oils, such as safflower, sunflower, corn, and soy. But omega-3 fatty acids are not as prevalent in our diet today.

Fish naturally contain the omega-3 fatty acids EPA and DHA, particularly the "fatty fish," like salmon, tuna, sardine, Chilean sea bass, trout, and the like. The parent omega-3 compound ALA is present in some plants, including algae, flaxseed, and chia seed. Our bodies can convert some of this ALA into EPA and, to a lesser extent, DHA.

Whole-body benefits of omega-3s

It is quite common to be deficient in omega-3s and supplementing with omega-3 fatty acids offers several benefits for our hearts, brains, and skin. Omega-3 supplements are also recommended for women who are trying to get pregnant or who are pregnant, as these good fats are essential to the growing brain, eyes, and nervous system of the baby.

Omega-3s and Heart Health

Several studies have evaluated the cardiovascular effects of omega-3 fatty acids. The majority of the research has focused on dietary consumption of fish and fish oil supplements. A few studies have also looked at the effects of the parent compound of the omega-3 family, ALA, but it appears that DHA and EPA are the most important omega-3s that have been proven to improve cardiovascular outcomes.

Omega-3s can support heart health in numerous ways: They reduce inflammation and clotting, significantly lower triglycerides (blood fats), and modestly raise HDL (good) cholesterol. They may also help reduce blood pressure, lower levels of homocysteine, reduce arrhythmias, and improve blood vessel tone.

Omega-3s and cardiovascular disease

The U.S. Department of Health and Human Services Agency for Healthcare Research and Quality conducted a review of the clinical research on omega-3 fatty acid supplements or fish consumption to assess the benefits on various cardiovascular disease (CVD) outcomes. This review involved 39 studies. Most of the large studies found fish consumption was associated with lower rates of all-cause mortality (death) and CVD outcomes (heart attack and stroke).[6]

Choosing an Omega-3 Supplement

Fish oil provides the highest amount of omega-3s of all supplements. Look for a pharmaceutical-grade, cold-pressed fish oil from a reputable manufacturer. If you cannot tolerate fish oils or prefer a vegetarian formula, take a supplement that provides omega-3 fatty acids from algae, chia seed, or flaxseed.

The American Heart Association recommends omega-3 fatty acids in capsule form (approximately 850 to 1000 milligrams [mg] of EPA and DHA) as an adjunct to the diet of women with heart disease, and higher doses — 2 to 4 grams — for women with high triglyceride levels.[7] Even higher dosages have been used in some studies — to match the dosage used in several major studies, you would need to take enough fish oil to supply about 2 to 3 grams of EPA and about 1.0 to 2.5 grams of DHA daily. Speak with your healthcare provider to determine what's best for you.

Omega-3 Precautions

Fish oil is generally well tolerated. The most common side effect that people report is fishy burps and, less commonly, upset stomach. Fish oil has a mild blood-thinning effect; however, it does not seem to cause bleeding problems when taken alone or with aspirin. There are a few isolated reports of it enhancing the blood-thinning effect of the drug warfarin (Coumadin, see Chapter 5). Nonetheless, people who are at risk of bleeding should consult with their doctor before taking fish oil.

One issue that has been raised with fish oil is purity. Many types of fish contain mercury, along with dioxins and PCBs — chemicals that are detrimental to health. However, according to U.S.-based Consumerlab.com, an organization that tests quality and label claims of nutritional supplements, this has not been a problem with most fish oil supplements because they are purified and tested for contaminants. Nonetheless, there is a prescription form of omega-3s, known as Lovaza (in the U.S.) or Omacor (elsewhere), and this is the most purified form of fish oil with the highest concentration of DHA and EPA currently available.

Supportive Supplements

Many supplements are promoted as offering benefits for heart health. Some of these products are backed by science, others by marketing hype. In this section we outline supplements that have been scientifically studied and shown to offer benefits. Beyond fish oil, none of these supplements has been shown to reduce heart disease outcomes (heart attack or stroke) or death. However, these supplements may help to manage some of the risk factors for heart disease — lowering blood pressure, cholesterol, or triglycerides, or reducing plaque formation, for example. If you are considering taking any of these supplements, consult with your doctor and pharmacist first and do not stop taking any of your prescribed medications.

Coenzyme Q10

Coenzyme Q10 (also known as ubiquinone, ubidecarenone, or simply CoQ10) is an antioxidant compound found in every cell in the body. It plays a vital role in the *mitochondria*, which is the powerhouse of the cell — the part that produces energy from glucose and fatty acids.

Research suggests that CoQ10 can support heart health, perhaps by helping it use energy more efficiently. A number of studies have shown it to be beneficial for treating congestive heart failure. It also offers modest benefits for blood pressure.

A brief history of CoQ10

Coenzyme Q10 was first discovered in 1957 by Professor Fredrick L. Crane and colleagues at the University of Wisconsin–Madison Enzyme Institute. The following year, Dr. Karl Folkers of Merck Pharmaceuticals identified and described the substance as coenzyme Q10, naming it "ubiquinone" because of its widespread — ubiquitous — presence in nature. Although Merck soon became disinterested, Dr. Folkers became increasing intrigued by CoQ10, pioneering scientific studies to determine its biochemistry and action. The Japanese were the first to test CoQ10 in humans. Today, CoQ10 is one of the top six most prescribed pharmaceutical agents in Japan.

CoQ10 Precautions

CoQ10 has a very good safety profile. There have been no reports of significant adverse side effects of oral CoQ10 supplementation at doses as high as 1,200 mg per day for up to 16 months and 600 mg a day for up to 30 months. Some people experience nausea, diarrhea, appetite suppression, heartburn, and abdominal discomfort while taking the supplement. These adverse effects may be minimized by dividing daily doses of more than 100 mg into two or three daily doses.

CoQ10 has been found to reduce blood sugar levels in people with diabetes. While this can be a beneficial effect, those with diabetes should monitor their blood sugar levels closely and be supervised by their doctor when taking CoQ10, as a change in medication may be required.

Taking CoQ10

Most of the research conducted with CoQ10 for heart health used daily dosages between 60 and 300 mg, although some studies have used much higher dosages. CoQ10 is a fat-soluble nutrient and is best absorbed with fats in a meal. Doses higher than 100 mg per day are generally divided into two or three doses throughout the day.

Garlic

Garlic has been used as a food, spice, and medicine for thousands of years. It is one of the most studied products for heart health. Yet research on the cardiovascular benefits of garlic has yielded mixed results. This may be in part because of the wide variety of garlic products tested — garlic oils, powders, macerates, and aged garlic extract — which vary greatly in their active compounds.

The most widely studied form of garlic is *aged garlic extract* (brand name Kyolic), which has been the subject of over 500 scientific papers. Aged garlic extract differs from other garlic supplements in that it is produced by extraction and aging of organic, fresh garlic, which eliminates the harsh and odor-causing compounds while retaining the beneficial compounds. Other garlic supplements that have undergone more limited clinical research are Kwai and Garlicin.

Aged garlic extract can offer modest benefits for lowering blood pressure, reducing cholesterol and triglyceride levels, lowering homocysteine levels, and reducing blood clotting. Preliminary research also suggests that aged garlic extract may slow the progression of plaque formation in the arteries, a process that can lead to heart disease or stroke.

Heart drugs may have serious interactions with herbal supplements such as ginkgo biloba, St. John's wort, and garlic. Always check with your doctor or pharmacist before taking any supplements.

Garlic Precautions

Garlic is generally safe and well tolerated. Some garlic supplements cause garlic breath and body odor, heartburn, and upset stomach. These side effects are uncommon with aged garlic extract.

Garlic can thin the blood, reducing its ability to clot, so it should not be taken before, during, or after surgery or if you have a bleeding disorder. Similarly, use it cautiously and under doctor supervision if you are taking blood-thinning drugs such as warfarin or clopidogrel (see Chapter 5), or herbal products with blood-thinning effects, such as ginkgo biloba. Studies evaluating the effects of aged garlic extract with oral anti-coagulants found no increase in bleeding.

Taking Garlic

The typical dosage of aged garlic extract is 600 to 1,200 mg daily with meals, but higher dosages have been used in some studies. The recommended dosage of dehydrated garlic (Kwai) is 2 tablets three times daily with meals. The recommended dosage for garlic powder (Garlicin) is 250 mg twice daily.

The great garlic debate

Over 100 compounds in garlic have been identified, and there is ongoing debate about which of these compounds are responsible for garlic's health benefits. Some manufacturers claim that allicin is the active compound, yet allicin cannot be measured in the blood or urine. When garlic is crushed or cut (or encapsulated), an enzyme called allinase is brought in contact with alliin, turning it into allicin. Allicin is responsible for much of garlic's odor and is an unstable compound that is broken down into a variety of other substances. Significant research has focused on other compounds in garlic, such as S-allyl cysteine, an antioxidant sulfur compound that can be measured in the body and has documented health properties.

Niacin

Also known as vitamin B3, or nicotinic acid, *niacin* has been used since the 1950s to improve cholesterol levels, and today it is an accepted mainstream treatment. Several studies have shown that niacin can raise levels of HDL cholesterol even better than prescription drugs like statins and can lower triglycerides. Niacin also helps lower LDL (bad) cholesterol, but to a lesser extent than it raises HDL (good) cholesterol. In some cases, niacin is prescribed along with statins or other cholesterol-lowering drug to increase the effects on LDL cholesterol.

Niacin has other heart-health benefits: it decreases levels of lipoprotein(a) and fibrinogen, which can reduce the risk of heart disease. However, niacin also increases homocysteine levels, which can increase this risk. Several studies have looked at the effects of niacin, alone and in combination with other drugs, for the prevention of heart disease and fatal heart attacks. Overall, this research suggests that niacin does provide benefits, especially when it is combined with other cholesterol-lowering drugs.[8]

Getting niacin through your diet

Niacin is found naturally in many foods, including yeast, meat, poultry, fish (tuna and salmon), milk, eggs, green vegetables, and cereal grains, although the amount present in foods is insufficient for lowering your cholesterol.

Niacin Precautions

Niacin in foods does not have any adverse effects. However, there are some precautions with the supplemental dosages used for lowering cholesterol. One main concern with niacin is that it can cause *flushing* reactions (warming and reddening of the face), especially at higher dosages. This can be annoying, especially if you are already experiencing hot flashes from menopause. The good news is that this reaction usually goes away over time. Niacin can also cause skin itching, upset stomach, and headache. More seriously, the use of niacin is associated with a risk of liver inflammation. This occurs more commonly with slow-release niacin.

Niacin can also interact with other cholesterol-lowering drugs. There are a few cases where the use of niacin with statin drugs may have caused *rhabdomyolysis*, a condition in which muscle cells are broken down, releasing enzymes into the blood and potentially causing kidney failure. For these reasons, the use of niacin requires close physician monitoring.

Taking Niacin

The recommended amounts of niacin range from 14 to 18 mg daily for adults, with a maximum intake of 35 mg daily. For cholesterol-lowering benefits, much higher dosages (1 to 6 grams of immediate release or up to 2 grams of extended release daily) are used.

Niacin supplements are available as nicotinic acid, nicotinamide, and inositol hexaniacinate. Only niacin (nicotinic acid) and nicotinamide have been studied thoroughly for cholesterol lowering. Nicotinamide is generally better tolerated than nicotinic acid, as it causes less flushing; however, it can still elevate liver enzymes and cause liver inflammation. It is claimed that inositol hexaniacinate is safer than ordinary niacin but there is no evidence to support this claim or any proposed benefits for cholesterol-lowering benefits.

Reduce flushing

To reduce the risk of facial flushing and upset stomach, take niacin after meals (never on an empty stomach) and start with a lower dose and gradually increase as directed. If you are taking niacin only once daily, take it with your evening meal. Taking aspirin 30 minutes before niacin can reduce flushing. Spicy foods may worsen the flushing. Avoid alcohol with niacin, as that may increase the risk of liver damage and worsen flushing. Nicotine (smoking) may also worsen flushing.

Phytosterols (Plant Sterols)

Phytosterols, the collective term for "phyto sterols" and "phyto stanols," are fat-like plant compounds with chemical structures similar to cholesterol. (*Stanols* are the saturated form of sterols.) The cholesterol-lowering effects of sterols were first observed in animals in the 1950s. Since then, a significant amount of research has shown that both sterols and stanols can help to lower cholesterol levels: studies show that consumption of phytosterols inhibits the intestinal absorption of cholesterol and reduces both total and LDL cholesterol levels.

The best dietary sources of phytosterols are vegetables, seeds, and nuts and their oils. Sterols and stanols are added to some margarine spreads, yogurt, and salad dressings, among other foods (you'll see this on the label), and also available as dietary supplements.

Phytosterol Precautions

Sterols are presumed safe because they are naturally present in many foods. Stanols are also considered safe because they are not absorbed into your bloodstream. No significant adverse effects have been reported in any of the studies that looked at the impact of sterols or stanols on lowering cholesterol. Because sterols reduce cholesterol absorption, it was thought that they may impair the body's absorption of fat-soluble vitamins; however, this is not an issue at the typical dosages used.

Taking Phytosterols

Although we consume phytosterols in our everyday diet, the amount is not sufficient to have a significant cholesterol-lowering effect. The FDA allows a heart-health claim for products that provide a minimum of 1.3 grams of sterol esters or 0.8 grams of sterols per day. Phytosterols need to be taken on a daily basis to provide any health benefits. The maximum effective dose for lowering LDL cholesterol is about 2 grams per day.

Various drinks, juices, margarine, salad dressings, yogurts, and other food products are now being fortified with phytosterols. Several supplements also contain sterols and are marketed for their cholesterol-lowering and heart-health benefits, including Centrum Cardio with CoroWise phytosterols.

See Chapter 8 for more on phytosterols.

Red yeast rice extract

Also known as Hong Qu, red yeast rice extract is a Chinese product that is used as a medicinal agent and food colorant. It is made by culturing a yeast on rice. This process produces compounds that have been purified and marketed as the drug lovastatin (Mevacor). While several studies have shown that red yeast rice can significantly reduce LDL cholesterol levels, it should be used cautiously and only under doctor supervision because it can cause serious side effects. According to a recent report, formulations of red yeast rice vary widely in their level of active ingredients and some may contain a toxin from fungus that is toxic to the kidneys.[9]

Phytochemicals

As discussed in Chapters 6 and 8, there is good evidence that a diet rich in vegetables and fruits offers many benefits for the heart. These benefits are attributed to *phytochemicals*, naturally occurring compounds found in plant foods. Many of these phytochemicals are developed into supplements for therapeutic use. Below we've listed some phytochemicals that may offer benefits for heart health. The research on these supplements is considered preliminary yet promising.

We must turn to nature itself, to the observations of the body in health and in disease to learn the truth.

— Hippocrates

Flavonoids

Flavonoids are a large family of compounds present in plants, including fruits and vegetables, which are associated with multiple health benefits. Flavonoid-rich foods include apples, berries, grapes (and wine), citrus fruit, tea, cocoa (yes, chocolate contains these compounds!), onions, and soybeans. Several studies have found that higher flavonoid intakes are associated with significant reductions in heart disease. The heart-health benefits of flavonoids are attributed to their antioxidant properties and their ability to reduce inflammation, promote relaxation of blood vessels, lower cholesterol levels, and reduce blood clot formation.

Numerous supplements containing flavonoids are available in health food stores and pharmacies. One product that appears to be helpful for lowering cholesterol levels is Sytrinol. Sytrinol is a patented formula that contains flavonoids and other antioxidants derived from citrus and palm fruit extracts. Preliminary research has shown that Sytrinol can lower total and LDL cholesterol and triglycerides. Sytrinol is well tolerated with no significant adverse effects. The recommended dosage is 300 mg daily.

Grape Seed Extract

The health benefits of grapes have received a great deal of attention, particularly because of the *French Paradox* — the low rate of coronary heart disease among the French despite a diet typically rich in saturated fats. It was thought that the low incidence of heart disease was linked to the relatively high consumption of red wine, and particularly to the polyphenolics found in grapes (more on this in Chapter 8). *Polyphenolics* are compounds highly concentrated in grape seeds and also present in the skin, pulp, and stem.

The heart benefits of grape seed extract, which contains *anthocyanins* — those polyphenolics that have red pigment — and is often a byproduct of winemaking, are tied to its ability to relax and open up blood vessels. One particular extract, available as Meganatural BP, has shown promise for the management of high blood pressure. Preliminary research shows that this extract can lower both systolic and diastolic blood pressure in those with elevated blood pressure without any adverse effects. The recommended dosage is 150 to 300 mg daily.

Lycopene

Lycopene is part of the carotenoid family of antioxidants. (*Carotenoids* are compounds related to vitamin A.) It is a bright-red pigment that is naturally present in tomatoes and other red fruits. Lycopene is the most common carotenoid in the human body, and it is one of the most potent carotenoid antioxidants.

The most widely studied lycopene supplement is Lyc-O-Mato, which provides a standardized amount of lycopene along with the other phytochemicals naturally present in tomatoes, such as phytoene, phytofluene, beta-carotene, and tocopherols. Preliminary studies have shown that this supplement can lower blood pressure in those with mild hypertension or moderate hypertension that is poorly controlled on medication. Lyc-O-Mato is well tolerated; no adverse effects have been reported in studies.

Research suggests, too, that lycopene as an antioxidant can inactivate free radicals, reduce LDL cholesterol, and slow the progression of atherosclerosis. Although more research is needed, it appears that lycopene offers heart-health benefits. And lycopene offers other potential benefits for women: some research suggests it has a protective effect against ovarian and breast cancer. It also protects the skin against sun damage.

Most research suggests consuming 10 servings of tomato products each week, which equals 6 to 15 mg of lycopene daily.

Overhyped: Folic acid and vitamin E

There are certain supplements that were thought to be beneficial for heart health yet have been proven otherwise. Two examples are folic acid and vitamin E. Folic acid (the synthetic form of folate added to foods or found in supplement form) was initially thought to be helpful because it is one of the B vitamins (along with B12 and B6) that helps lower homocysteine levels (see Chapter 2), and high homocysteine levels are associated with heart disease. However, clinical studies evaluating the effects of folic acid on heart health have found that it either doesn't offer benefits or can actually be harmful. With vitamin E, studies conducted many years ago suggested that it may help reduce heart disease risk, yet more recent research has not found it to be beneficial. Heart failure can result from several causes, including a heart attack or coronary artery disease (where one or more of the coronary arteries is narrowed), hypertension, valve disorders, chemotherapy drugs, alcohol, or infections or disease processes that affect the heart muscle.[10]

Selecting and Taking Supplements

There are many factors to consider when choosing and taking supplements and certain precautions to keep in mind. Here are some tips:

♥ Research your options. Look for products that are backed by scientific studies. The list of resources at the end of this book will point you toward organizations that provide consumer-friendly information about supplements.

♥ Consult with your doctor, pharmacist, or healthcare provider and find out as much as you can about the supplement you are considering taking. Even if they are not familiar with the product, they can access and interpret scientific information about the product. In particular ask if there are any possible interactions with medications or side effects.

♥ If you are pregnant, nursing, have a chronic medical condition, or plan to have surgery, be sure to consult with your healthcare provider before taking any supplements.

♥ Read the labels carefully. Look for an expiration date and make sure the product is well within that date. If there is no expiration date on the label, don't buy it.

♥ Don't choose a supplement based on price. A more expensive product does not necessarily mean it is better. Some vitamins are more expensive because of company marketing and advertising costs, not because of higher-quality ingredients. Conversely, however, cheaper products may be filled with additives and lower-quality ingredients.

♥ Avoid supplements with chemical additives (*excipients*) such as talc, corn, wheat, dairy, artificial flavorings and colorings (dyes), and preservatives, unless no alternative is available. These are unnecessary ingredients that can cause allergic reactions in some people.

♥ Call the manufacturer if you have questions about a certain brand.

♥ Buy from a reputable manufacturer. Ask your pharmacist or health food store adviser for a recommendation.

♥ Don't stop taking a prescribed drug or substitute a supplement for a prescribed drug unless under the advice and supervision of your healthcare provider.

♥ Take the supplements regularly. With some, such as fish oils, you may not notice a difference in how you feel, but they are working and need to be taken consistently for you to reap the benefits.

♥ Don't take a higher dosage of a product than is recommended on the label unless your healthcare provider advises you to do so.

♥ Don't continue to take a supplement if you have a bad reaction, such as prolonged upset stomach or rash or anything unusual.

Nature, time and patience are the three great physicians.

— Bulgarian proverb

The Heart of the Matter

Nutritional supplements can play an important supportive role in heart health. Certain supplements can help reduce risk factors for heart disease such as high blood pressure and cholesterol, clotting, and inflammation. The evidence is strongest for omega-3 fatty acids, which have been shown to actually reduce the incidence of heart attack and stroke. As researchers continue to study the effects of nutrients and herbs, we will learn more about the role of these products in disease prevention and treatment.

Keep in mind that although these products are seen as "natural," that does not mean that they are safe and without side effects. Always speak with your healthcare provider before taking any new product and never stop taking a medication or replace a medication with a natural product unless your physician advises you to do so.

Chapter 8

Heart Bites

You are what you eat . . .
— Your mother

Yes, the quotation that opens this chapter is a cliché that we have all heard before, but it is absolutely true. We often don't think very much about what we are putting into our bodies, yet our dietary choices have a significant impact on our heart and overall health. Poor dietary choices, such as eating foods that are high in saturated fat, trans fats, sugar, and salt, compromise our well-being. Even if you don't have heart disease now, these food choices will catch up with you later and eating them can pave the way to disease. On the other hand, making the right dietary choices can promote good health.

Hippocrates said it wisely: "Let food be thy medicine."

Food provides our body with energy, nourishment, and a range of nutrients that can protect against disease. We now know that certain foods and ways of eating can be as powerful as medicine; they can help to reduce the risk of heart disease and other chronic health problems and play a role in treating disease.

Over the past few decades, numerous dietary approaches have been promoted to improve heart health. (When we use the word "diet," we are referring to a way of eating, rather than a weight-loss diet.) Most healthful diets recommend eating fruits, vegetables, lean protein, and whole grains, and limiting unhealthy fats (saturated and trans fats). These choices are considered the dietary essentials for good health. Various dietary approaches have emerged as research has uncovered the dangers of certain foods — saturated fat, trans fats, sugar, high-glycemic carbohydrates, excess sodium — and the benefits of other foods — olive oil, fish, tomatoes, red wine — to heart health. In this chapter we provide a brief overview of some of the recommended diets for heart health and who may benefit from following these approaches. We share with you our philosophy on nutrition and heart health, give you information on our top recommended foods for your heart and those you should avoid, and explore some nutritional myths and controversies.

The DASH Diet

The typical North American diet can contain a whopping 3,500 milligrams (mg) of sodium (salt) or more a day — way more than your body needs. High sodium intake is linked to high blood pressure (*hypertension*), a risk factor for heart attack, among other serious health problems. The DASH (Dietary Approaches to Stop Hypertension) diet is a dietary approach designed to help treat or prevent high blood pressure. It encourages reducing sodium intake and eating a variety of foods rich in nutrients such as potassium, calcium, and magnesium that help lower blood pressure.

There are two versions of the DASH diet. The standard DASH diet allows up to 2,300 mg of sodium a day. The lower-sodium DASH diet allows up to 1,500 mg of sodium a day. Studies show that the lower-sodium DASH version is especially helpful in lowering blood pressure in adults who are middle-aged or older, in African Americans, and in those who already have high blood pressure.

Both versions of the DASH diet include lots of whole grains, fruits, vegetables, and low-fat dairy products, as well as fish, poultry, and legumes. Red meat, sweets, and fats are allowed in small amounts. This diet is low in saturated fat, cholesterol, and total fat. It recommends reducing your sodium intake by using sodium-free spices or flavorings with food instead of salt; not adding salt when cooking rice, pasta, or hot cereal; rinsing canned foods to remove as much of the sodium as possible; and buying foods labeled "no salt added," "sodium free," "low sodium," or "very low sodium."

Normal blood pressure in a healthy young adult is 120/80 mmHg (units of millimeters of mercury) or lower. Blood pressure consistently higher than 140/90 mmHg is considered to be high. Studies show that the DASH diet can lower blood pressure by a few mmHg in just two weeks. Over time, your blood pressure could drop by 8 to 14 mmHg, which can make a significant difference in your health risks. If you add exercise and weight loss to the DASH program and restrict alcohol (one or fewer drinks a day for women) you can potentially reduce your blood pressure by 21 to 55 mmHg.

Glycemic Index Diet

With this dietary approach, the *glycemic index* (GI) guides your food choices. The GI is a scale ranging from zero to 100 that ranks carbohydrate-rich foods by how fast they raise blood sugar levels compared with a standard food, usually pure glucose, which is ranked at 100.

Generally, foods that are low in soluble fiber and more processed will break down quickly and have a high GI rating (70 and above). Such food are white bread, white rice, cookies, many breakfast cereals and bars, baked potatoes, and sugary drinks. Foods that break down slowly have a low GI rating (55 or less). Most vegetables, high-fiber whole grains (like wild rice and steel-cut oats), sweet potatoes, and many fruits, including berries, apples, and citrus fruit, fall into this category. Foods with a GI ranking of 56 to 69 are considered to have a moderate GI and they include sweeter fruits like mango and pineapple and some starchy vegetables like corn and potatoes (boiled or mashed). The GI diet is not a low-carb or no-carb diet. This diet advocates choosing quality foods (low to moderate GI carbs) and minimizing your intake of high-GI foods.

High-GI foods are problematic because they are rapidly digested (broken down into sugar), triggering a rapid rise in blood sugar and insulin levels. When your blood sugar and insulin levels stay high, or cycle up and down rapidly, your body has trouble responding to the changes and, over time, you may develop insulin resistance. *Insulin resistance* is associated with a host of health problems, including type 2 diabetes, obesity, and heart disease. High-glycemic meals are thought to increase the risk of heart disease by increasing triglycerides (blood fats) and cholesterol, promoting inflammation, and impairing blood vessel function.

The lesser of two evils

A recent landmark study published in The American Journal of Clinical Nutrition *reported that refined, highly processed carbohydrates are worse for your heart than saturated fat. This study revealed that replacing saturated fat with refined carbohydrates actually puts you at greater risk for heart attack than not avoiding saturated fats. Researchers compared the association between saturated fat and carbohydrates with the risk of heart attack among 53,644 healthy individuals over a 12-year time period. Substituting some carbohydrate in the diet with saturated fat did not alter the likelihood of heart attack. However, replacing some saturated fat in the diet with high-GI carbohydrate boosted the risk of heart attack by 33%.*[1]

The GI diet is not a new concept. Many popular diets are based in part on the glycemic index, including Nutrisystem, the Zone Diet, and Sugar Busters. A low-GI diet was initially thought to be most beneficial for improving blood sugar control in diabetics, but recent research has shown that it can also help people in general with weight loss and heart disease prevention.

The Mediterranean Diet

Long before the Mediterranean diet became well known in North America, this way of eating was natural for folks living around the Mediterranean Basin, namely Spain, Italy, and Greece. Researchers observed the lower incidence of chronic diseases, like heart disease and cancer, among people in this region and key patterns in their diets and lifestyles. Key components of the Mediterranean diet include:

♥ eating a generous amount of fruits and vegetables
♥ consuming healthy fats such as olive oil and canola oil
♥ using herbs and spices instead of salt to flavor foods
♥ eating nuts, in small portions
♥ drinking red wine, in moderation, for some
♥ consuming very little red meat
♥ eating fish or shellfish at least twice a week
♥ getting plenty of exercise
♥ eating your meals with family and friends

Several studies have found that the Mediterranean diet helps lower LDL (bad) cholesterol. This diet is ideal for those with heart disease or those aiming to prevent heart disease.

The American Heart Association Diet

The American Heart Association has developed an eating plan to prevent heart attack and stroke, another cardiovascular disease. It includes the following recommendations:

♥ Eat a variety of vegetables and fruits (five servings per day).
♥ Eat a variety of grains (six servings per day).
♥ Eat fish at least twice a week, preferably fatty fish such as salmon and tuna.
♥ Choose legumes, skinless poultry, lean meats, and reduced-fat dairy products.
♥ Select fats with no more than 2 grams of saturated fat per tablespoon — liquid and tub margarine, and canola, corn, safflower, and olive oils.
♥ Limit high-calorie, low-nutrient foods like soft drinks and candy.
♥ Limit foods high in saturated fat, trans fat, and cholesterol.
♥ Maintain sodium intake to 2,400 mg or 1 1/4 teaspoons per day.
♥ Limit alcoholic beverages to no more than one drink per day for women.

In addition to reducing risk factors for heart disease, this plan can help with weight loss and improve other aspects of health.

Our Philosophy: A Balanced Approach

The diets we've outlined share many common features: they emphasize fruits, vegetables, whole grains, and healthy fats, and they recommend minimizing saturated fat (such as that in red meat), refined/processed foods, and salt.

But you won't find us touting any special heart-health diet. We are not advocates of strict dieting programs or ways of eating that make you feel deprived. And, quite frankly, we don't like the word "diet" because it often evokes a feeling of restriction. As well, many people see diets as a short-term way of eating. We believe that proper nutrition is integral for good health and that this has to be part of your lifestyle. We believe in a healthy, reasonable approach to eating that focuses on eating satisfying foods that provide your body and your heart with the essential vitamins, minerals, essential fatty acids, and nutrients required for optimal health. So rather than give you strict dietary rules to follow, we suggest these general guidelines:

♥ Eat three meals and two snacks daily — or rather, five small meals. Small, frequent meals keep your energy levels high, promote better blood sugar control, and reduce hunger and cravings for not-so-healthy foods.

♥ Boost your fiber and nutrient intake by eating lots of fruits, vegetables, beans, and whole grains.

♥ Eat more foods that offer specific benefits for heart health such as berries, fish, garlic, nuts, and soy foods. The specific benefits of and research on these foods are discussed in this chapter.

♥ Drink lots of water and green tea.

♥ Minimize processed and fast foods, as they are typically high in calories and have little nutritional value. These foods are also high in saturated and trans fat, sugar, and salt — all detrimental to heart health. We discuss these issues later in this chapter.

♥ Watch your portion sizes. This is where many of us go astray. For example, a serving of grains equals one slice of bread or 1/2 cup of cooked rice, pasta, or cereal. Yet many restaurants serve pasta portions that are equivalent to three or four servings. The U.S. and Canadian governments have issued dietary guides detailing the recommended number of servings of each food category per age group and what constitutes a serving. Visit www.mypyramid.gov or http://www.hc-sc.gc.ca for details.

If, however, you have concerns beyond heart health, such as weight loss or diabetes management, you may want to choose a particular dietary approach to meet your goals. For example, if you are concerned about heart disease and are also trying to lose weight and improve your blood sugar control, you may want to follow the GI diet. If you have hypertension, you may want to follow the DASH diet.

Heart-Healthy Foods

As you know by now, dietary choices have a significant impact on the health of your heart. Certain foods can help reduce cholesterol levels and provide you with essential fatty acids, vitamins, minerals, and other nutrients that support heart health. In fact, what you eat is just as important as what you don't eat (which we cover later in this chapter). In this section we outline our top heart-healthy foods. Aim to incorporate lots of these foods into your daily diet.

Legumes

Beans (also called *legumes*) provide a significant amount of soluble fiber, which can help lower cholesterol levels. In fact, one cup of cooked beans provides between 9 and 13 grams of fiber. Beans are also a good source of protein, complex carbohydrates, and B vitamins. The nutritional content of most dry beans is very similar, with the exception of iron: white beans have almost twice the iron of black beans, whereas kidney beans are somewhere in between. On the other hand, black beans are a particularly good source of antioxidants, followed by red, brown, yellow, and white beans.

Several studies have evaluated the heart-health benefits of legumes. In one large study, researchers examined the effects of legumes on various forms of cardiovascular disease, including heart disease and stroke, by studying 19 years of data gathered from 9,632 people in the United States who participated in the National Health and Nutrition Examination Survey I Epidemiology Follow-Up Study. Participants were between the ages of 25 and 74 when the study began and were free of cardiovascular disease. They were divided into several groups: those who ate beans less than once per week, those who ate beans once per week, those who ate beans two or three times per week, and those who ate beans at least four times per week. The study found that legume consumption four times or more per week, compared with less than once a week, was associated with a 22% lower risk of coronary heart disease and an 11% lower risk of all forms of heart disease.[2]

Beans are a great addition to soups, stews, salads, and dips. Rinse dry beans well with lukewarm water before cooking. To shorten their cooking time, presoak beans in cool water for several hours to rehydrate them, changing the soaking water at least once. This gets rid of some of the gas-causing compounds and makes the beans easier to digest.

Berries

These tiny little fruits burst with flavor, are powerful sources of nutrition, and provide benefits for various aspects of health, including heart health. They provide us with many vitamins (especially vitamins C and E) and fiber, and they rank low on the glycemic index.

The beautiful blue, purple, and red colors of berries are due to naturally occurring pigments called *anthocyanins*. These compounds belong to the flavonoid family of antioxidants and have been the subject of a number of studies. (Cherries, grapes, and red wine are also good sources of anthocyanins.) Anthocyanins improve the integrity of support structures in the blood vessels, reduce stickiness of platelets (platelets are tiny blood cells that play a key role in clot formation, and platelet aggregation or "stickiness" is linked to heart attack), raise HDL levels, and inhibit free-radical damage and inflammation.

Cranberries for heart health

Of all the berries, cranberries have the most research supporting heart health. Studies suggest that cranberry juice (one to two 8-ounce glasses per day) can help raise HDL (good) cholesterol and lower LDL (bad) cholesterol and triglyceride levels. Cranberries have also been shown to reduce oxidation of LDL cholesterol (a precursor to atherosclerosis) and improve blood vessel function.

Blackberries, blueberries, cranberries, raspberries, and strawberries are the most popular berries. But more and more, lesser-known berries such as goji and açaí are gaining attention as their health benefits are explored. To get the most nutritional impact from berries, choose fresh or frozen berries, as canned, dried, or processed berries have significantly lower levels of antioxidants.

Chia Seed

The chia plant (*Salvia hispanica*) has a rich history of use in ancient cultures. In pre-Columbian civilizations, such as that of the Aztecs, chia seeds were used as a high-energy food and were a staple of the daily diet. In the 1980s, the plant gained notoriety thanks to a catchy TV commercial jingle for the chia pet. We don't recommend eating chia from your chia pet; instead, check at your health food store for chia seed that is grown and cultivated for human consumption.

The wonder seed

Chia seeds are an excellent source of protein, calcium, fiber, vitamins, and minerals. They actually provide a higher level of antioxidants than fresh blueberries. Chia oil — available bottled or in gel capsules — is one of the richest plant sources of omega-3 fatty acids. The seeds are naturally gluten-free, low in the glycemic index, and most are produced through organic farming.

Chia seeds provide about 41 grams of dietary fiber per 100-gram serving — about one-fourth of which is soluble fiber — making them a perfect food for a heart-healthy lifestyle. Foods high in soluble fiber — fiber that dissolves in water and, once consumed, beneficially slows the rate of digestion and absorption — can help lower cholesterol levels and may reduce the risk of heart disease. Research suggests that chia can reduce after-meal blood glucose levels, which is an important feature for diabetics and weight management. One small preliminary study compared the effects of chia seed to wheat bran in a group of diabetics. Those who consumed 37 grams (4 teaspoons) of chia seed per day over a 12-week period experienced a significant decrease in HbA1c (measure of blood glucose control) and a modest reduction in systolic blood pressure. Levels of C-reactive protein, a key marker of inflammation, fell 30%, and clotting factors dropped 20%. Levels of both plasma ALA (alpha-linolenic acid) and eicosapentaenoic polyunsaturated fatty acid (an omega-3 fatty acid) were increased twofold in those consuming chia seed.[3] (Read more about these beneficial fatty acids in Chapter 7.)

Adding chia to your diet

Add a tablespoon or two of chia seed to your cereal, yogurt, or smoothie, or incorporate chia into recipes for breads and other baked goods. To make chia gel, add a tablespoon of chia seeds to 1/2 cup water, stir, let stand five minutes, then stir again. The seeds absorb about 10 times their weight in water, creating a thick gel that can be used as a thickener for dressings, sauces, jellies, or smoothies.

Cinnamon

Cinnamon is one of the oldest known spices. The characteristic flavor and aroma of cinnamon come from essential oils naturally present in the bark. In traditional Chinese medicine and *Ayurveda*, an ancient Hindu healing art, cinnamon is used for colds, stomach complaints, diabetes, and to improve energy and circulation.

Research suggests that cinnamon may have benefits for heart health, particularly in those with diabetes. Several small preliminary studies have found that cinnamon can modestly improve blood glucose and cholesterol levels. In one of the first human studies, 60 people with type 2 diabetes took 1, 3, or 6 grams of cinnamon in pill form daily, an amount roughly equivalent to 1/4 teaspoon to 1 teaspoon of cinnamon. After 40 days, all three amounts of cinnamon reduced *fasting blood glucose* (blood glucose after a fast of about eight hours — commonly used to measure glucose levels) by 18 to 29%, triglycerides by 23 to 30%, LDL cholesterol by 7 to 27%, and total cholesterol by 12 to 26%.[4]

Cinnamon may have some blood-thinning effects, particularly in large amounts, so people who take blood thinners should consult with their doctor before adding cinnamon to their diet. Because of its effects on blood sugar, diabetics should also be cautious about consuming cinnamon and have their blood sugar levels checked when they do.

Adding cinnamon to your diet

Cinnamon is a great addition to homemade baked goods such as cookies, cakes, and muffins. Sprinkle it on cereal, oatmeal, yogurt, and baked apples, incorporate it into smoothies, or add it to your next curry.

Fish

Fish has become one of the most highly recommended foods for heart health because it is a good source of omega-3 fatty acids and protein and it is low in saturated fat. Omega-3 fatty acids can benefit not only those with heart disease but also those who are healthy but at risk of heart disease. Research shows that omega-3 fatty acids decrease the risk of *arrhythmias* (abnormal heartbeats), which can lead to sudden death. Omega-3 fatty acids also decrease triglyceride levels, slow the growth rate of atherosclerotic plaque, reduce the risk of blood clots, and have a modest effect on lowering blood pressure. Studies show that in people who have already had heart attacks, fish oil or omega-3 fatty acids can significantly reduce the risk of sudden death.

Those who don't like eating fish or are unable to get adequate amounts of omega-3s through their diet might consider taking a fish oil supplement. Other food sources of omega-3s include chia seed, flaxseed, and algae. Omega-3 supplements are discussed further in Chapter 7.

Put fish on your weekly menu

The American Heart Association recommends eating two servings of fish, particularly fatty fish, once per week.[5] Each serving is 3.5 ounces cooked, or about 3/4 cup of flaked fish. Fatty fish like salmon, mackerel, herring, lake trout, sardines, and albacore tuna are high in omega-3 fatty acids. People with high triglycerides can benefit from taking higher amounts of fish oil than it is practical to get through diet alone — omega-3 supplements or prescription omega-3 fatty acids (Lovaza) may be necessary.

Mercury, PCBs, and Fish

The health benefits of fish are well documented. Unfortunately, there is some bad news. Fish contains mercury and chemicals known as PCBs, which are associated with various adverse health effects.

Mercury occurs naturally in the environment and can also be released into the air through industrial pollution. Mercury accumulates in streams and oceans, where it is turned into methylmercury. Fish absorb the methylmercury as they feed in these waters, and it can build up in their bodies. Methylmercury can be harmful to the developing nervous system of an unborn baby and young child. Nearly all fish and shellfish contain traces of mercury, but some have higher amounts, depending on what they eat. Fish that have lived longer and are higher on the food chain have the highest levels of methylmercury because they've been accumulating it longer.

The Food and Drug Administration and the Environmental Protection Agency (EPA) advise women who may become pregnant, pregnant women, nursing mothers, and young children to avoid some types of fish and eat fish and shellfish that are lower in mercury. Here are the specific recommendations:

♥ Do not eat shark, swordfish, king mackerel, or tilefish, which contain high levels of mercury.

♥ Eat up to 12 ounces (two average meals) a week of a variety of fish and shellfish that are lower in mercury. Five of the most popular fish that are low in mercury are shrimp, canned light tuna, salmon, pollock, and catfish. Another commonly eaten fish, albacore (white) tuna, has more mercury than canned light tuna. When choosing your two weekly meals of fish and shellfish, limit your intake of albacore tuna to 6 ounces (one average meal).

♥ Check local advisories about the safety of fish caught by family and friends in local lakes, rivers, and coastal areas. If no advice is available, eat up to 6 ounces (one average meal) per week of fish caught in local waters, but don't consume any other fish during that week.[6]

Polychlorinated biphenyls (PCBs) are another concern. Exposure to these synthetic organic chemicals is associated with harmful effects on health. Although PCBs are no longer manufactured in North America, people can still be exposed to them through the environment, workplace, and the consumption of fish.

Recent studies indicate that susceptible populations (certain ethnic groups, sport anglers, the elderly, pregnant women, fetuses, nursing infants, and children) continue to be exposed to PCBs through fish and wild-game consumption and this exposure can have deleterious effects on health. Studies indicate that (1) reproductive function may be disrupted by exposure to PCBs; (2) neurobehavioral and developmental deficits occur in newborns and continue through school-aged children who were exposed to PCBs in utero; (3) other systemic effects (self-reported liver disease and diabetes, and effects on the thyroid and immune systems) are associated with elevated blood levels of PCBs due to exposure/ingestion; and (4) increased cancer risks, including of non-Hodgkin's lymphoma, are associated with PCB exposures.[7]

PCBs build up in fish and animal fat, so certain cooking methods can help reduce your exposure:

♥ Before cooking, remove the skin, fat (found along the back, sides, and belly), internal organs, and the tomalley of lobster and the mustard of crabs, where toxins are likely to accumulate.
♥ When cooking, be sure to let the fat drain away and avoid or reduce fish drippings.
♥ Serve less fried fish; frying seals in chemical pollutants that might be in the fish's fat; grilling or broiling allows fat to drain away.
♥ For smoked fish, fillet the fish and remove the skin before the fish is smoked.

The U.S. Environmental Defense Fund, based on EPA guidance and the latest mercury and PCB data, recommends limiting consumption of certain fish, including striped bass, eel, bluefin tuna, flounder, and salmon, because of elevated PCB levels.[8]

Garlic

Garlic has a long history of use as a medicine. Many ancient civilizations, for example the Greeks, Egyptians, and Romans, used garlic to increase strength. In Taoism, it is believed that garlic enhances one's *chi* energy, or vital life energy. In Ayurveda, garlic is described as a medicinal plant used to bring warmth to the body as well as to improve blood circulation.

Research has looked at the role of garlic in heart health (more on this in Chapter 7). Garlic contains powerful sulfur-containing compounds, including *thiosulfinates* (such as *allicin*), *sulfoxides* (*alliin*), and *dithiins* (*ajoene*), that are responsible for its pungent odor. These compounds are also the source of many of its health-promoting effects. Garlic is a good source of manganese, vitamins B6 and C, and selenium.

Garlic's healing power

Several studies have shown that garlic may play a modest role in helping to lower total and LDL cholesterol, as well as triglycerides. It can help reduce oxidation of cholesterol and slow the progression of atherosclerosis. Garlic also helps reduce blood clotting, relax blood vessels, and slightly lower blood pressure.

The American Dietetic Association has suggested that to obtain the potential health benefits of garlic, one must consume 600 to 900 mg (about one fresh clove) per day. For optimal flavor and nutritional benefits, consume fresh garlic. Garlic flakes, powders, or jarred sliced garlic may be more convenient but do not offer the same nutritional and health benefits as fresh. When buying garlic, look for bulbs that are plump and with unbroken skin. Avoid garlic that is soft, moldy, or that has begun to sprout, which may indicate decay.

Green Tea

Tea has been a popular beverage for thousands of years, but only in the past few decades have researchers studied its health benefits. Green tea is made from the *Camellia sinensis* plant. Black and oolong teas are also made from this same plant. These teas differ in how they are processed. Green tea is the least processed and so provides the most antioxidant polyphenols, notably a catechin called *epigallocatechin-3-gallate* (EGCG), which is responsible for many of green tea's health benefits.

Numerous studies have found that green tea drinkers have lower rates of several diseases, including cancer, heart disease, stroke, periodontal disease, and osteoporosis. Research suggests that green tea can protect against heart disease in many ways. It helps lower LDL cholesterol, triglycerides, *lipid peroxides* (free radicals that damage LDL cholesterol and other lipids or fats), and *fibrinogen* (a protein in the blood involved in the formation of blood clots), while improving the ratio of LDL to HDL cholesterol. Green tea catechins help thin the blood and prevent the formation of blood clots by preventing pro-inflammatory compounds from forming. Some evidence suggests that green tea can help lower blood pressure. Research also shows that green tea catechins inhibit the enzymes involved in the production of free radicals in the endothelial lining of the arteries. The *arterial endothelium* is a one-cell-thick lining that serves as the interface between the bloodstream and the wall of the artery — where plaque can form.

Green tea: Antioxidant powerhouse

An 11-year study involving 40,530 adults examined the association between green tea consumption and death due to all causes, cardio-vascular disease (CVD), and cancer. Compared with participants who consumed less than one cup of green tea per day, those who drank five or more cups a day had a significantly lower risk of death from all causes and, specifically, risk of death from CVD, with women receiving even stronger protection than men. Women had a 23% lower risk of dying from any cause and a 31% lower risk of dying from all forms of cardiovascular disease. They also looked at specific forms of cardiovascular disease, and women who consumed five cups of green tea daily had a 42% and 62% lower risk of death due to stroke and cerebral infarction, respectively. For men the risk reduction was 12%, 22%, and 42%, respectively. Only weak or neutral relationships were seen between black tea or oolong tea and death from all causes or from CVD.[9]

Green tea is certainly one of the healthiest beverages you can drink, particularly for your heart. Most of the research showing the health benefits is based on the amount of green tea typically consumed in Asian countries — about three cups per day, which would provide 240 to 320 mg of polyphenols. Green tea does contain caffeine, but much less than coffee does. One cup of green tea contains about 20 to 45 mg of caffeine; decaffeinated green tea is also available. There are many types of green tea to choose from, including those from China, Japan, and India, and they vary greatly in both quality and price. Visit a specialty tea shop to explore and sample the wide range available.

Oats

Oats are one of the most highly recommended foods for heart health because they provide more soluble fiber than any other grain. The type of soluble fiber in oats, called *beta-glucans*, has been shown to help lower cholesterol. Soluble fiber offers other benefits, too: it helps slow digestion and absorption of food and promotes a feeling of fullness, and it helps improve blood glucose levels. Oats are also a great source of manganese, selenium, vitamin B1, magnesium, phosphorus, and protein.

Oats' health claim

More than 40 clinical studies conducted over the past few decades have shown oats' ability to fight heart disease. The evidence is so significant that the Food and Drug Administration (FDA) allows a health claim to be made on the labels of foods containing soluble fiber from whole oats (oat bran, oat flour, and rolled oats), noting that 3 grams of soluble fiber daily from these foods, in conjunction with a diet low in saturated fat and cholesterol, may reduce the risk of heart disease. To qualify for the health claim, the whole oat–containing food must provide at least 0.75 grams of soluble fiber per serving.[10]

Whole grains such as oats may be particularly beneficial for postmenopausal women with high cholesterol and heart disease. A three-year study of over 200 postmenopausal women with heart disease, published in the *American Heart Journal*, shows that those who ate at least six servings of whole grains each week experienced slowed progression of atherosclerosis and less progression in *stenosis* (the narrowing of the diameter of arterial passageways). The women's intake of fiber from fruits, vegetables, and refined grains was *not* associated with a lessening in cardiovascular disease progression.[11]

Three grams of soluble fiber from oats daily is equivalent to about 1 1/2 cups of cooked oatmeal. You can further boost the fiber of your oatmeal by adding berries, bananas, flax or chia seed, or dried fruit.

Olive Oil

This famous oil from the Mediterranean is rich in monounsaturated fat, a type of fat that offers various health benefits. The popularity of olive oil has soared in recent years as several epidemiological (population-based) studies have found significantly lower rates of death from all causes, particularly heart disease, among those whose dietary habits are closest to traditional Mediterranean diets — rich in plant foods and olive oil and low in saturated fats. Not only does olive oil contain good fats but it also offers a potent mix of antioxidants, including vitamin E, carotenoids, and polyphenolic compounds.

Olive oil's health claim

The FDA allows this health claim for olive oil: "Eating about 2 tablespoons (23 grams) of olive oil daily may reduce the risk of coronary heart disease due to the monounsaturated fat in olive oil. To achieve this possible benefit, olive oil is to replace a similar amount of saturated fat and not increase the total number of calories you eat in a day."[12]

Studies show that olive oil can help lower your LDL cholesterol while leaving your HDL cholesterol untouched. A review of clinical studies by noted olive oil researcher Maria Covas strongly suggests that diets in which olive oil is the main source of fat can be useful against a wide variety of risk factors for cardiovascular disease. According to Covas, "The benefits of olive oil consumption are beyond a mere reduction of the LDL cholesterol."[13]

Research suggests that olive oil helps reduce inflammation and oxidation of cholesterol and protect against atherosclerosis. Adding olive oil to your diet may also help protect against clot formation and even lower blood pressure, particularly in those with high blood pressure.

Some reports suggest that the cholesterol-lowering effects of olive oil are even greater with extra-virgin olive oil. *Extra-virgin olive oil* is derived from the first pressing of the olives and has the most delicate flavor and the most antioxidant benefits. It may cost more, but you reap more health benefits and taste. Avoid "light" olive oils. This label usually means the oil has been more processed and is lighter in color, not lighter in fat or calories.

Adding olive oil to your diet

There are lots of ways to incorporate olive oil into your diet. Add olive oil to breads, potatoes, and other vegetables instead of butter. Use it in salad dressings, dips, and marinades. To get the most health benefit and flavor from your olive oil, buy and store oil in opaque glass containers and add olive oil to foods immediately after cooking — heating the oil will diminish its flavor and nutritional value.

Phytosterols (Plant Sterols)

Phytosterols, the collective term for phyto sterols and phyto stanols, are fat-like substances that occur naturally in many vegetables, fruits, nuts (cashews, pistachios, pecans, and walnuts), and seeds (pumpkin, sesame, and sunflower). They are added to certain foods and are also available in supplement form.

As mentioned in Chapter 7, phytosterols have been found to lower both total and LDL cholesterol, while not affecting the levels of the HDL cholesterol. They work by blocking the absorption of cholesterol. Studies show that foods and drinks fortified with phytosterols can help reduce LDL cholesterol by more than 10%. They do, however, interfere with the absorption of the fat-soluble vitamins — vitamins A, D, E, and K.

Phytosterols' health claim

The evidence on phytosterols is so significant that the FDA allows a heart-health claim for products containing a certain level of sterols or stanols: Foods containing at least 0.65 g per serving of plant sterol esters (or 1.7 g per serving of plant stanol esters), eaten twice a day with meals for a daily total intake of at least 1.3 g of sterols (or 3.4 g of stanols), as part of a diet low in saturated fat and cholesterol, may reduce the risk of heart disease.[14]

Drinks, juices, margarine, salad dressings, yogurts, and other food products are now often fortified with phytosterols. Here are some examples:

♥ CoroWise phytosterols by Cargill are found in a growing number of foods and beverages, such as Minute Maid Premium Heart Wise, Rice Dream Heartwise, and Kroger Active Lifestyle milk.

♥ Unilever offers Promise Activ Light Spread with phytosterols in the United States.

♥ Astro in Canada now offers Astro BioBest Plant Sterols yogurt.

You need to take phytosterols on a daily basis to reap their benefits. The maximum effective dose for lowering LDL cholesterol is about 2 grams per day. This is equivalent to about two 8-ounce (237 milliliters) servings of phytosterol-fortified orange juice a day. Keep in mind that phytosterol food products still contain fat and calories — just because a product contains phytosterols does not mean that you should eat unlimited amounts.

Soybeans

Soybeans have been a staple in the Asian diet for thousands of years. This legume is popular for its nutty flavor and exceptional nutritional value. Like other beans, soybeans grow in pods; the seeds, which can be green, yellow, brown, or black, are edible.

Soybeans are an excellent source of protein. One half-cup serving (about 4 ounces) of firm tofu provides about 10 grams of protein and 5 grams of fiber, along with iron, magnesium, omega-3 fatty acids, isoflavones and other nutrients. Soy is naturally cholesterol-free and low in saturated fat. This makes the soybean a valuable alternative to animal proteins, which are higher in saturated fat and lower in nutritional value.

The soybean is one of the most well researched health foods, offering benefits for the heart, bones, menopause management, and cancer prevention. For heart health, studies have shown that it can help lower total cholesterol levels by 30% and LDL levels by as much as 35 to 40%. Some studies show it also helps raise HDL cholesterol levels and lower triglycerides and reduce blood pressure. Soy helps reduce the "stickiness" or clumping of platelets, which reduces the risk of blood clots. Soy protein protects against atherosclerosis, too, by increasing blood levels of *nitric oxide*, a chemical that improves blood vessel dilation and inhibits *oxidative* (free radical) damage of cholesterol and the adhesion of white cells to the vascular wall. These are all important factors in the development of atherosclerosis.

Soy's health claim

The evidence on soy is so significant that in 1999 the FDA approved a health claim for soy protein. The claim states that "25 grams of soy protein a day, as part of a diet low in saturated fat and cholesterol, may reduce the risk of heart disease."[15]

A meta-analysis of 23 studies published from 1995 to 2002 which appeared in *The American Journal of Clinical Nutrition* reported that consumption of soy protein, with its isoflavones intact (as in soy foods) resulted in decreases in total cholesterol by 3.77%, LDL cholesterol by 5.25%, and triglycerides by 7.27%, plus increases in HDL cholesterol by 3.03% — all significant amounts. Studies in which participants consumed more than 80 mg of soy protein daily resulted in better effects on the *lipid profile* (a group of tests to measure triglycerides and LDL, HDL, and total cholesterol, to determine a person's risk of heart disease). Tablets containing extracted soy isoflavones did not produce a significant effect on total cholesterol reduction.[16]

Soy and Breast Cancer

Many population-based studies indicate that women with diets high in soy have lower rates of breast cancer, yet the safety of consuming soy has been questioned because soy contains isoflavones, which are phyto-estrogens (plant-based estrogens), and estrogen (hormone replacement therapy) has been found to increase breast cancer risk. It is important to realize that soy isoflavones have only one-thousandth the potency of human estrogens and most research has shown that they actually have anti-estrogenic activity by blocking estrogen at its receptor sites. While some animal studies have found that soy may stimulate breast cancer cells in certain circumstances, there is no convincing evidence that consuming moderate amounts of soy (levels typical in an Asian diet) increases the risk of breast cancer in healthy women or worsens the prognosis of women with breast cancer.[17]

For optimal health, eat whole soy foods — edamame, whole soy flour, tofu, and tempeh — rather than eating processed soy products or taking soy supplements. Be aware that tofu does contain some saturated fat. For example, a half-cup serving (4 ounces) of firm tofu contains a total of 4 grams of fat, of which 0.5 grams is saturated fat. Generally, the softer the tofu, the lower the saturated fat.

Adding soy to your diet

Add soybeans to soups, stews, salads, and dips. Soy flour can replace wheat flour when making breads, muffins, and other baked goods.

Tomatoes

Tomatoes contain a compound called lycopene, which belongs to the carotenoid family of antioxidants. Lycopene is twice as powerful as beta-carotene and offers a range of health benefits for the heart, skin, and more. (Read more about this in Chapter 7.)

Heart-healthy lycopene

The heart benefits of lycopene are thought to be tied to its ability to reduce total and LDL cholesterol levels, lower blood pressure, fight free-radical damage and inflammation, and reduce blood clotting. In addition to lycopene, tomatoes are a very good source of other heart-healthy nutrients such as potassium and a good source of niacin, vitamin B6, and folate.

Several population studies have suggested that consuming lycopene-rich tomato products can help lower the risk of heart disease. Research conducted at Brigham and Women's Hospital, Boston, MA, tracked close to 40,000 middle-aged and older women who were free of heart disease when the study began. During more than seven years of follow-up, those who consumed seven to ten servings each week of lycopene-rich foods (tomato-based products, including tomatoes, tomato juice, tomato sauce, and pizza) were found to have a 29% lower risk of cardiovascular disease compared to women eating less than one and a half servings of tomato products weekly. Women who ate more than two servings each week of oil-based tomato products, particularly tomato sauce and pizza, had an even better result — a 34% lower risk of heart disease.[18]

Another study, published in *The American Journal of Clinical Nutrition*, further highlighted the benefits of lycopene for women. This 4.8-year study, involving almost 40,000 middle-aged and elderly women in the Women's Health Study, found that as the women's blood levels of lycopene went up, their risk for cardiovascular disease dropped. Study subjects were divided into four groups in order of increasing blood levels of lycopene. A 34% reduction in cardiovascular disease risk was seen in women in the top two groups, but even women in the second highest group were still 22% less likely to develop cardiovascular disease compared to women in the lowest group. After excluding women with angina, those whose plasma lycopene levels were in the three highest groups were found to have a 50% reduced risk of cardiovascular disease compared to those with the lowest blood levels of lycopene.[19]

Add tomatoes to salads, soups, stews, sandwiches, and dips, and use them to make sauces, tomato paste, ketchup, and salsa. To get the most lycopene from your tomatoes, use the whole tomato, including the antioxidant-rich skin.

Five Foods You (and Your Heart) Will Love

If the previous list of foods didn't excite your taste buds, you will be pleased to read about our five favorite foods that not only taste good but are also good for your heart. These indulgent foods are often surrounded by misconceptions, so put aside what you may have heard about them and read on. We can help you justify your love of these foods, so you can enjoy them without feeling guilty.

Avocados

Avocados are fruits (actually large berries) that grow on trees throughout much of the world — particularly in Mexico, the Caribbean, and Central and South America. Avocados often get a bad rap because they are high in fat. However, the primary type of fat this fruit provides is the beneficial kind, namely monounsaturated fat. A small (100-gram/3.5-ounce) avocado provides 9.8 grams of monounsaturated fat and only 2.13 grams of saturated fat. Mono- and polyunsaturated fats, when consumed in moderation and eaten in place of saturated or trans fats, can help reduce blood cholesterol levels and decrease risk for heart disease. Avocados are one of the few fruits that provide "good" fats. Avocados are also a good source of protein, fiber (both insoluble and soluble), phytosterols, B vitamins, folic acid, and vitamins E and K. Plus, avocados provide 60% more potassium than bananas.

Avocados are part of the Mediterranean diet discussed earlier in this chapter, which has been shown to be beneficial for heart health. One short-term study evaluated the impact of an avocado-rich diet in a group of healthy people and a group with elevated cholesterol levels. Total cholesterol levels declined in both groups after just seven days of consuming an avocado-rich diet. Those with high cholesterol experienced the most benefits: a 17% decrease of *serum total cholesterol* (the level of total cholesterol in the blood), a 22% decrease in LDL cholesterol and triglycerides, and an 11% increase of HDL cholesterol.[20]

Avocados also promote healthy skin and hair. Although they can be found in skincare products, they are likely most beneficial when eaten rather than applied directly to your hair or skin.

Choosing an avocado

The skin of a ripe avocado is typically dark green or greenish-brown or black. If it is bright green, it isn't ripe. You can also tell if it is ripe by its firmness: Hold the avocado in the palm of your hand and apply gentle pressure to the ends — a ripe avocado will yield slightly with gentle pressure when squeezed at the ends. The flesh is typically greenish-yellow to golden-yellow when ripe. Once an avocado is cut and exposed to air, it turns brown quickly. To prevent this — particularly desirable when adding avocado to salads or making dips like guacamole — squeeze lime or lemon juice over the sliced avocado.

Chocolate

Chocolate is made from seeds of the tropical *Theobroma cacao* tree. Its popularity as a beverage and ingredient in foods dates back over 1000 years. The Aztecs treasured it as a decadent treat, referring to it as the "food of the gods." Chocolate is a favorite of many folks (including us!) and it is estimated that the average person consumes about 11 pounds (5 kilograms) of chocolate per year.

Chocolate and your heart

Chocolate not only tastes delicious but also offers a wealth of health benefits. The antioxidant flavonoids in cocoa help reduce the risk of clotting and protect the inside lining of arteries that feed the heart. Cocoa has been shown to reduce LDL cholesterol and modestly reduce high blood pressure. Some chocolate products now have phytosterols added, which boosts their heart benefits.

A recent study published in *The American Journal of Clinical Nutrition* looked at the impact of various flavonoid-rich foods on the risk of heart disease and mortality over a 16-year period in a group of 34,489 postmenopausal women participating in the Iowa Women's Health Study. They found that women who consumed the most flavonoid-rich food had a 22% lower risk of developing heart disease. Chocolate was ranked as one of the top flavonoid-rich foods associated with a protective effect, along with bran, red wine, grapefruit, and strawberries.[21]

Another recent study looked at whether consuming chocolate could reduce incidence of heart failure among women. This nine-year study involved 31,823 women, ages 48 to 83, with no history of diabetes, heart failure, or myocardial infarction. The researchers found that women who consumed a moderate amount of chocolate (one to two servings per week) were less likely to have heart failure compared to those who reported no regular intake of chocolate.[22]

To obtain the most benefits from chocolate, reach for dark chocolate. The more chocolate is processed, the fewer flavonoids it retains, meaning it has fewer potential health benefits. Dark chocolate has the most flavonoids, almost four times as many as milk chocolate. White chocolate isn't truly chocolate — it is not made with cocoa and does not contain any flavonoids. Rather, white chocolate contains primarily sugar and fats. Choose dark chocolate that contains at least 70% cocoa (cocoa solids or cocoa mass will be listed first on the ingredients list, not sugar or milk ingredients). Dark chocolate is still a source of calories, fat, and sugar, so enjoy it in moderation. While a few small pieces of dark chocolate daily can be good for you, eating a full chocolate bar every day may very well lead to weight gain — not good for your heart.

Is chocolate an aphrodisiac?

Chocolate has long been associated with love. In the Mayan and Aztec cultures, the cocoa bean was considered an aphrodisiac. Today, chocolate is considered an ideal gift for a lover. And there just might be a scientific explanation for the loving feelings we get when we eat chocolate. Chocolate provides a high amount of the chemical phenylethylamine, which is capable of raising dopamine levels in the brain. Dopamine is a chemical messenger (neurotransmitter) involved in our feelings of pleasure.

Coffee

Many of us rely on a cup of coffee to jumpstart our day — this aromatic beverage helps awaken the mind and the senses. Coffee is prepared from roasted coffee seeds (beans) that come from the coffee cherries that grow on the coffee plant — typically shrubs or small trees. It is thought that coffee drinking originated in Ethiopia centuries ago and then spread to Yemen, Egypt, Arabia, and the rest of the world. Today, coffee is one of the most popular beverages worldwide and grown in more than 70 countries.

Coffee contains various compounds, including caffeine and antioxidants. Over the past few decades there have been numerous reports on the potential health benefits and risks associated with drinking coffee. On the positive side, some research has suggested that coffee can reduce the risk of dementia, Alzheimer's disease, Parkinson's disease, type 2 diabetes, and cirrhosis of the liver. Some of these effects are linked to the caffeine and others to the antioxidant compounds.

High amounts of caffeine can raise blood pressure, and some research suggests that drinking caffeinated coffee can cause a temporary increase in the stiffening of arterial walls. But here is the good news: coffee also contains a significant amount of antioxidants, which are beneficial for heart health. A recent review concluded that habitual coffee drinking was associated with a lower risk of coronary heart disease in women.[23] In this review, researchers examined data from 21 studies and reported that moderate coffee consumption (of up to four cups of coffee per day) was associated with an 18% reduction in risk of heart disease in women.

Another recent study, published in *Circulation*, suggested that coffee consumption may protect women against stroke.[24] In this report, researchers analyzed data from a group of 83,076 women in the Nurses' Health Study without history of stroke, coronary heart disease, diabetes, or cancer. Coffee consumption was assessed first in 1980 and then repeatedly every two to four years, with follow-up through 2004. The researchers found that compared with women who drank less than one cup of coffee a month, the risk of all types of stroke was:

♥ 20% less in women who drank four or more cups/day
♥ 19% less in women who drank two to three cups/day
♥ 12% less in women who drank coffee five to seven cups a week

Other drinks containing caffeine, such as tea and caffeinated soft drinks, were not associated with a benefit for stroke.

Coffee conundrum

Some of the mixed reports about the heart-health effects of coffee could be due to the way coffee is prepared. Coffee prepared using paper filters (drip coffee) removes oily components called diterpenes that are present in coffee. These diterpenes have been associated with increased risk of coronary heart disease due to elevation of LDL levels in the blood. Metal filters, on the other hand, do not remove diterpenes from the coffee, so for people using a French press or percolator or who drink espresso, a cholesterol check may be in order.

Because of its caffeine content, coffee can have a stimulating effect and should be avoided or consumed conservatively if you have insomnia, anxiety, or a stress disorder. It can also worsen acid reflux. Pregnant women should moderate their intake of caffeine to 200 mg per day from all sources (coffee, tea, chocolate, and soft drinks) because of increased risk of miscarriage. Coffee can interfere with iron absorption, so don't consume it along with your multivitamin or iron supplements.

Did you know . . .

♥ The average coffee drinker consumes 3.1 cups of coffee per day.

♥ Black coffee with no sugar or cream or milk has no calories.

♥ Drinking a single cup of coffee that has been brewing for 20 minutes provides the body with 300 phytochemicals, which act as antioxidants and stay in the body for up to a month.

♥ Espresso coffee has just one-third of the caffeine content of ordinary coffee.

♥ Caffeine increases the effect of some painkillers such as aspirin and paracetamol (acetaminophen), which is why it is often an ingredient in pain medications.

Nuts

Many of us avoid nuts because we hear they are high in calories and fat. Yet almonds, walnuts, pistachios, and hazelnuts, for instance, contain many heart-healthy compounds, including monounsaturated fat, phytosterols, L-arginine, magnesium, potassium, and antioxidants such as vitamin E. Nuts are also a good source of protein and fiber.

Of all the nuts, almonds and walnuts have the most research supporting their cholesterol-lowering benefits. Several studies have shown that nuts can significantly reduce blood cholesterol and help keep blood vessels healthy and elastic. A review of studies linking nuts and a lower risk of coronary heart disease was published in the *British Journal of Nutrition*. Researchers looked at four large studies: the Adventist Health Study, Iowa Women's Study, Nurses' Health Study, and the Physicians' Health Study. When evidence from all four studies was combined, subjects who consumed nuts at least four times a week showed a 37% reduced risk of coronary heart disease compared to those who never or seldom ate nuts. Each additional serving of nuts per week was associated with an average 8.3% reduced risk of coronary heart disease.[25]

Although nuts are high in calories, some studies have found that increasing nut consumption by several hundred calories per day (i.e., a handful of nuts) does not cause weight gain. In a study published in the journal *Obesity,* researchers found that people who ate nuts were much *less* likely to gain weight. The 28-month study involving 8,865 adults found that participants who ate nuts at least two times per week were 31% less likely to gain weight than were participants who never or almost never ate nuts.

This doesn't mean you can enjoy endless amounts of nuts. Here, too, moderation is the key. Replace other foods high in saturated fat with nuts. For example, instead of putting cheese, meat, or croutons in your salad, add a small handful of nuts (about 10 almonds) or have a tablespoon of almond or cashew butter on your toast instead of regular butter. Nuts are also a nice addition to cereal, yogurt, and steamed vegetables. Choose unsalted nuts to avoid spiking your sodium intake.

Nuts' health claim

In July 2003, the FDA approved the first qualified health claim specific to nuts lowering the risk of heart disease: "Scientific evidence suggests but does not prove that eating 1.5 ounces (42.5 g) per day of most nuts, as part of a diet low in saturated fat and cholesterol, may reduce the risk of heart disease."[26]

Red Wine

You have likely heard about the heart-health benefits tied to red wine. This is welcome news to wine enthusiasts who like to sip a glass of wine without feeling guilty. Over the past few decades, several studies have demonstrated that moderate consumption of wine is associated with a decrease in death caused by heart disease.[27] A lot of the research has focused on red wine, as it is a particularly good source of antioxidant compounds, including polyphenols, flavonoids, and resveratrol. These compounds help to raise HDL cholesterol and prevent platelets in the blood from sticking together, reducing the risk of clot formation and heart attack or stroke. Some of these benefits may be found in other foods such as red and white grapes or red-grape juice.

Interest in the health benefits of red wine exploded with the theory of the *French Paradox* — the comparatively lower incidence of heart disease in France despite high levels of saturated fat in the traditional French diet. It has been thought that this association is due to the relatively high consumption of wines by the French. However, there are some researchers who suggest that other factors may be at play, as some studies have found that the average moderate wine drinker is also more likely to exercise more, to be more health conscious, and to be of a higher socioeconomic class.

It is important to note that the benefits of drinking wine (and other alcohol) are tied to a moderate intake: one drink per day for women (in contrast to 1-2 drinks per day for men). A drink is 12 ounces of beer, 4 ounces of wine, 1.5 ounces of 80-proof spirits, or 1 ounce of 100-proof spirits. Drinking too much alcohol can raise triglycerides and also contribute to high blood pressure and heart failure. Alcohol also floods the body with empty calories, and excessive calorie intake can lead to obesity and increased risk of diabetes. For these reasons, the American Heart Association does not recommend drinking wine or any other form of alcohol to gain the heart benefits. So the bottom line is that if you enjoy drinking wine, do so in moderation.

Red or white?

Red wine has a higher concentration of antioxidants, particularly resveratrol, which are associated with the cardio-protective benefits. Resveratrol is present in the skins and seeds of the grape, used when fermenting the grape juice during the red wine–making process. This prolonged contact during fermentation produces significant levels of resveratrol in the finished red wine. White wine contains resveratrol too, but the seeds and skins are removed early in the process, reducing the concentration of the compound in the finished white wine.

Nutritional Heart Breakers

Now that we have talked about all the foods that are good for our hearts, we must discuss those that are not so good, as well as others that are downright dangerous for our hearts and our health.

Trans Fatty Acids

Trans fatty acids, also know as trans fats, are found in hydrogenated oils, which are present in some margarines, baked goods, snack foods, and deep-fried foods (e.g., French fries). Even microwave popcorn often contains hydrogenated oils. These fats can raise cholesterol levels and increase the risk of heart disease. Choose non-hydrogenated margarines and look for snacks labeled as having no trans fats. Many snack food companies are now making products that are free of trans fatty acids.

Saturated Fat

Saturated fat, present in animal foods and certain oils, can raise cholesterol and triglyceride levels and is associated with increased heart disease risk. Foods high in saturated fat include meat, poultry with skin, seafood, and high-fat dairy products (milk, cheese, butter, cream, whipped cream, ice cream, and sour cream). Vegetable oils and margarine also contain some saturated fat but much less than that found in animal products. Choose lean cuts of meat and limit the amount of beef you eat. Limit your consumption of saturated fat to 7% of your total daily calories.

Choosing low-fat dairy

It is best to choose low-fat dairy products over higher-fat ones, but be aware that the calorie count may be similar to that of products with a higher fat content. When manufacturers reduce the amount of fat, they often add sugar and/or starch. For example, low-fat and fat-free sour cream contains about the same number of calories. As well, dairy products labeled "low fat" may still have a substantial amount of fat. For example, 25% of calories in 2% milk come from fat. The "2%" refers to the fraction of volume filled by fat, not the percentage of calories coming from fat.

Cholesterol

Although saturated fat is the main culprit in high blood cholesterol levels, experts also caution against consuming too much dietary cholesterol. So limit foods that are high in dietary cholesterol, like organ meats, whole-milk products, and egg yolks. Aim for no more than 300 mg of dietary cholesterol daily. One egg yolk, for example, contains 213 mg cholesterol, so it is okay to eat a whole egg a day. Egg whites do not contain any cholesterol and are a good source of protein, so enjoy omelets and scrambled eggs made with egg whites.

Sugar and Refined Starches

Foods high in sugar and refined starches (white bread and baked goods) rank high on the glycemic index: they raise triglyceride and insulin levels and increase the risk of insulin resistance and risk factors for heart disease. Limit your intake of candy, cookies, and other sweets; choose whole grains (whole-grain bread and pasta, brown rice) over refined starches.

> *Eating a large, indulgent dinner that is high in fat and carbohydrates can constrict blood vessels, increasing the risk of blood clots.*

Salt

Salt causes water retention and increases the pressure inside the arteries. For most people, reducing salt intake reduces blood pressure. Aim to consume no more than 2,400 mg of sodium daily. Avoid adding salt to foods and minimize eating processed and fast foods such as deli meats, snacks (chips and pretzels), French fries, and burgers. Look for low-salt versions of soups, sauces, salad dressings, dips, crackers, and other foods.

One-quarter of what you eat keeps you alive. The other three-quarters keeps your doctor alive.
— Hieroglyph found in an ancient Egyptian tomb

Nutritional Controversies

We are constantly bombarded with mixed messages about food and nutrition. We hear conflicting information about the health effects of eggs, butter, artificial and natural sweeteners, and many other foods. Here we address common nutritional controversies, especially those that affect your heart, and we provide you with the bottom line on what you need to know.

The Egg Debate

Egg yolks contain dietary cholesterol, and eating eggs has been shown in most studies to raise blood cholesterol levels. However, the only large study to look at the impact of egg consumption on heart disease — not on cholesterol levels or other intermediaries — found no connection between the two. Some studies have shown that eating eggs may not even raise blood cholesterol if the overall diet is low in fat. Eating foods high in saturated fat has a greater effect on cholesterol levels, and an egg contains only 1.5 grams of saturated fat.

Bottom line: If you like eggs, eat them in moderation (one daily) and reduce your dietary intake of saturated fat.

Sea Salt or Table Salt?

Sea salt and table salt have the same basic nutritional value. Both consist primarily of the same amount of two minerals — sodium and chloride. Sea salt is often marketed as a more natural and healthy alternative, but the real differences between sea salt and table salt are in their taste, texture, and processing. Sea salt is produced through the evaporation of seawater, which leaves behind a small amount of trace minerals and elements that add flavor and color to sea salt. Table salt is mined from underground salt deposits. Table salt is more heavily processed to eliminate trace minerals and usually contains an additive to prevent clumping. Most table salt also has added iodine, an essential nutrient that appears naturally in minute amounts in sea salt.

Bottom line: Sea salt and table salt contain the same amount of sodium, so it is a matter of taste preference. But be aware that table salt is our primary source of iodine, so if you cut table salt out of your diet, you could become iodine deficient. Limit your salt intake to 1 1/4 teaspoon or 2,400 mg daily.

Diet versus Regular Soft Drinks

A regular-sized 12-ounce soft drink contains the equivalent of 9 teaspoons of sugar, usually in the form of high-fructose corn syrup, which has been linked to several health problems — obesity, type 2 diabetes, high blood pressure, and heart disease.

In an effort to cut calories and sugar, many people turn to diet soft drinks. However, diet soft drinks are loaded with chemicals like caffeine, artificial sweeteners (aspartame), sodium, and phosphoric acid that are not good for our health. Recent research suggests that artificial sweeteners may impair our body's sense of sugar satisfaction and reduce satiety, increasing hunger and cravings. Aspartame is also a neurotoxin and linked to migraines and many other adverse health effects.

Bottom line: Avoid both regular and diet soft drinks. These beverages don't provide any nutritional value and are potentially detrimental to health.

> *In the United States, 23% of Caucasian women, 38% of African American women, and 36% Mexican American women are obese. Obesity leads to an increased risk of premature death due to cardiovascular problems like hypertension, stroke, and coronary artery disease.*

Natural Sweeteners

In recent years there has been mounting interest in natural sweeteners like stevia and agave, but are these products good choices?

Stevia is an herb, and its extract can be up to 300 times sweeter than sugar with virtually no calories. Stevia's taste has a slower onset and longer duration than that of sugar. Stevia has been used as a sweetener in many parts of the world for several years. It is particularly popular with diabetics because it doesn't raise blood sugar levels and it may actually improve glucose tolerance. There is some evidence that stevia can help reduce blood pressure in those with hypertension. Some stevia products have a bitter or licorice-like aftertaste at high concentrations. Stevia appears to be safe in moderate doses. Side effects of stevia, such as nausea and a feeling of fullness, are generally mild.

Agave nectar (also called agave syrup) is a sweetener commercially produced in Mexico from several species of agave plants. In recent years, agave nectar has been promoted as a healthy sugar alternative because it is about one and a half times sweeter than sugar and is said to be natural. It has also been promoted as a safe sweetener for diabetics, but there is little evidence to support this claim. Agave nectar consists primarily of fructose and glucose, in varying amounts depending on the manufacturer and how it is processed. Some products contain as much as 92% fructose and 8% glucose. Raw agave nectar's glycemic index is comparable to fructose, which is lower than sugar (sucrose).

Here are the concerns with agave: Unless the product label states that the agave is raw, most agave syrup is harvested and processed using chemicals that transform it into a product more closely resembling high-fructose syrup, which is associated with adverse health effects. Agave syrup is not low calorie. In fact, it has about the same amount of calories per teaspoon as white sugar — approximately 16 calories. Depending on the source and how the nectar is processed, it may not be low on the glycemic index. Some manufacturers may add corn syrup to the agave nectar, further compromising the proposed health benefits.

Bottom line: If you are looking for a natural, calorie-free sweetener, consider stevia. Otherwise use sugar in moderation.

Butter versus Margarine

There is a long-standing debate on this one. Butter and margarine contain about the same amount of calories; however, butter, as an animal fat, contains both saturated fat and cholesterol. Saturated fats can raise LDL cholesterol and total blood cholesterol levels.

When margarine was first introduced it was thought to be a healthier alternative to butter because it is made from vegetable oils. However, to make liquid oil solid, a process called *hydrogenation* was used. This created trans fatty acids, which later were found to be very bad for our health. Trans fats can raise LDL cholesterol levels. In recent years, food manufacturers have created non-hydrogenated margarine, which contains no trans fat. Some margarines are also fortified with phytosterols, beneficial for heart health because they help lower cholesterol levels. You will also see heart-healthy omega-3 fatty acids added to some products.

Bottom line: Choose a non-hydrogenated margarine with added phytosterols, like Becel, Benecol, or Promise, or sparingly use a whipped butter or light or calorie-reduced butter — these have less fat and fewer calories because they have vegetable oils added.

Palm Oil and Coconut Oil

Palm oil and coconut oil are edible plant oils derived from the fruits of palm trees. Because these oils are high in saturated fats, and saturated fat can raise cholesterol levels and is associated with increased risk of heart disease, they have been thought to be not as healthy as other vegetable oils. Yet, what is more important is the balance of the fatty acids — unsaturated (polyunsaturated and monounsaturated) versus saturated — in a particular oil.

Palm oil contains about equal proportions of saturated and unsaturated fats and is particularly high in cholesterol-lowering polyunsaturated fatty acids. Palm oil is also a nutrient-dense oil containing many potent antioxidants including beta-carotene — a precursor of vitamin A — and tocotrienols — a potent form of vitamin E.

Several studies have shown that there is no significant rise in serum cholesterol when palm oil is used as an alternative to other fats in the diet. In fact, palm oil may have a beneficial effect on cholesterol levels, raising HDL cholesterol levels while having a neutral to beneficial effect on LDL cholesterol levels. Many food companies have replaced the hydrogenated oils (a source of trans fatty acids) in their products with palm oil.

There are other health benefits associated with the tocotrienols in palm oil. Emerging evidence suggests that tocotrienols can reduce the risk of stroke. Ground-breaking research conducted at Ohio State University by Dr. Chandan K. Sen has shown that Malaysian palm oil–source tocotrienols target specific pathways to protect against neural cell death and rescue the brain after stroke injury.[28] This particular source of tocotrienols, called Tocomin (made by Carotech Inc.) was used in all of the Ohio State University and National Institutes of Health–funded research conducted by Dr. Sen.

What makes Malaysian palm oil somewhat different from other oils is its high content of polyunsaturated fatty acids — the most of all the saturated fats (about five times more than coconut oil or butter fat). By contrast, palm kernel oil (like coconut oil) comes from the fruit's seeds and contains 85% saturated fatty acids and only 2% polyunsaturated fatty acids.

The more health-conscious food producers are using palm oil, which is relatively solid at room temperature yet contains sufficient polyunsaturates and monounsaturates to melt naturally into a liquid form when consumed. Unlike other oils, it doesn't need to be hydrogenated to work well in most processed food applications. As such, palm oil is often added to cookies and baked goods and spreads. One product that is widely available is Smart Balance HeartRight Buttery Spread, which contains Malaysian palm oil along with phytosterols and other healthy oils (fish and olive).

Coconut oil has also been given a bad rap because of its high content of saturated fat. Although coconut oil contains less polyunsaturated fat than palm oil, there is some recent evidence that pure/virgin coconut oil may actually have a favorable effect on cholesterol levels, raising HDL cholesterol. If using coconut oil, choose a virgin/pure form. Avoid hydrogenated or partially hydrogenated forms of coconut oil, as they contain trans fats.

Both palm and coconut oil are heat stable, which makes them ideal for cooking and baking at high temperatures.

Bottom line: Non-hydrogenated palm oil and coconut oil can be included as part of a healthy diet, but aim to keep your total daily fat intake between 25 and 35% of the calories you consume.

The Heart of the Matter

Science has clearly shown us that food can be as powerful as medicine and plays a strong role in disease prevention. This is particularly true when it comes to heart health. As you learned in this chapter, certain foods can help reduce cholesterol and blood pressure and reduce your risk of heart disease.

For your heart's sake, and for your overall health, aim to incorporate more of the heart-healthy foods we've discussed into your daily diet. Experiment with new recipes and be mindful of what you put in your mouth.

Neither of us are advocates of strict dieting. We all have our favorite foods and get accustomed to a particular way of eating. But keep in mind that our daily habits matter far more than an occasional indulgence. So focus on following a heart-healthy lifestyle rather than a restrictive diet and make the best possible choices for your heart.

Chapter 9

Exercise and Your Heart

Give a girl the correct footwear and she can conquer the world.
— Bette Midler

We agree with Ms. Midler that, given the right pair of shoes, we can conquer the world. And sometimes, the correct footwear is a pair of running shoes! Women need to be more active to save their hearts. We all have lots of reasons why we don't exercise, but it is time to cast those aside, dust off our running shoes, and get busy moving our bodies.

Exercise plays a critical role in preventing heart disease and it can even help to improve your health if you already have heart disease. In this chapter, we will talk about physical activity and physical fitness (they mean slightly different things), the benefits to your heart, how much is recommended, and how you can build more activity into your day.

Why We Need to Move

Our society is increasingly sedentary. You may be surprised to know that the majority of women report that they do not perform any physical activity on a regular basis; therefore, the majority of women do not meet the current recommendations for physical activity (we show you the recommendations later in this chapter). What this has translated to is a society that is increasingly overweight or obese. Currently two out of every three women are either overweight or obese, and these levels are increasing all over the world.

We are becoming more and more inactive, with our workdays getting longer and our jobs requiring more sitting than moving, using cars rather than our feet to get around, and spending a large amount of recreational time sitting in front of computers and televisions. In the 1950s, 50% of all jobs required physical activity, compared with about 25% of jobs today. As a result of inactivity, we are not only gaining too much weight, but all modifiable risk factors for heart disease are on the rise; we are now even more likely to have diabetes, hypertension, and high cholesterol. And the younger we are when we start reducing our daily physical activity, the earlier these risk factors can start developing, so we are shifting the onset of heart disease to occur in younger and younger women. We have to stop this trend now.

The *single most important* thing you can do for your heart is to be active and remain active throughout your life. Physical activity and physical fitness are essential for maintaining your heart, as well as your overall health. Physical inactivity is second only to cigarette smoking as the leading cause of preventable deaths and is positioned to take over and become the leading cause of preventable deaths. We can stop that from happening. We just need to move!

The Difference between Physical Activity and Physical Fitness

Lack of activity destroys the good condition of every human being, while movement and methodical physical exercise save it and preserve it.
— Plato

We talk about physical activity and physical fitness sometimes as if they were the same thing. They are most definitely related, but physical activity is a self-reported event, that is, far more *qualitative* (meaning more descriptive than measurable). If you're asked what activity you do, you might say you play tennis for 30 minutes a day, so it's clear you are active for that time, but it's not entirely clear how much energy you exerted when you played. It can be estimated, but it is not as precise as directly measuring it. On the other hand, physical fitness is more *quantitative*, meaning your level of fitness can be measured or estimated from your level of activity. For example, if you say you run 1 mile in 10 minutes, your level of fitness can be gauged. You can get on a treadmill or bicycle and perform a stress test, which quantifies your maximum fitness level by seeing what maximal speed and degree of incline (if a treadmill is used) or resistance (if a bicycle is used) you can tolerate. But the way physical activity and physical fitness are related is that the more physically active you are, the greater your physical fitness level.

Physical fitness is a measure of the highest work intensity that can be achieved with any given activity. It is measured in *metabolic equivalents*, also known as METs. A metabolic equivalent is a measure of the amount of oxygen required for any physical activity. Machines like treadmills, bicycles, and elliptical and rowing machines typically provide an estimate of the MET level you are at while working out; this will vary with the intensity of your workout. Most people usually just look at the machines to see the time they have worked out and calories they've burned, but it is also worthwhile to check your physical fitness level in METs. Recent research done by one of this book's authors, Martha, shows that a woman's physical fitness level, as measured on a traditional exercise stress test, is an independent predictor of mortality and cardiovascular mortality. This means that if you are not very physically fit, you have a greater chance of dying from any cause, and you have a particularly high risk of dying from cardiac causes.[1,2]

The inability to perform more than 5 METs places women at the highest risk of death, compared with women who can perform 8 METs or more. Martha and her research team also developed an equation to predict fitness level based on age (since we know fitness declines with age) and found, using a group of almost 6,000 women who were without symptoms of heart disease, that a woman's age-predicted fitness level is best determined by this equation:

$$\text{Age-predicted METs} = 14.7 - (0.13 \times \text{age})$$

Plugging your age into this equation will tell you what your 100% age-predicted fitness level should be. For example, if you are 51 years old, 100% of your age-predicted fitness level is 14.7 − (0.13 X 51) = 8 METs. The table below shows what your age-predicted fitness level should be at certain ages.

Age-Predicted Fitness Level

Age (years)	Metabolic Equivalents (METs)
30	11
40	9.5
50	8.2
60	7
70	5.6
80	4.3
90	3

We found that for women with or without cardiac symptoms, the inability to achieve 85% of that number was associated with a greater risk of death from cardiac causes, in addition to predicting an earlier death from any cause.[3] This study was published in *The New England Journal of Medicine* in 2005 and was ground-breaking research for women. Until that point, women had not been studied, and so there were no standard values established for physical fitness in women. Such values had been established in men, and despite knowing that women's fitness levels were different from men's, the equation for men was used for women. The value of measuring and knowing a woman's level of physical fitness appeared to be as important as other traditional cardiac risk factors in predicting her risk of heart disease.

How do you translate METs to your daily activities? Well, 1 MET is the amount of oxygen required to lie at a resting state, so any physical activity requires more fitness than that, and will be at least greater than 1 MET (with the exception of being sedentary, watching television, or sitting at the computer). Below is a list of common activities and the level of fitness required for each.

Activity	Physical fitness level (METs)
Watching television	1
Playing a musical instrument	2
Walking slowly (1–2 miles/1.5–3 kilometers per hour)	2
Golfing (using a cart)	3
Bowling	3
Fishing	3
Gardening	3–4
Leisure biking (less than 10 miles/16 kilometers per hour)	4
Dancing (moderate pace)	4
Golfing without a cart	5
Walking briskly (4 miles/6 kilometers per hour)	5
Tennis (doubles, not too intense)	5
Jogging (5 miles/8 kilometers per hour)	6
Rowing	6–8
Running (6 miles/9.5 kilometers per hour)	10
Swimming (moderately fast)	6–10
Tennis (singles)/Squash	8–12
Skiing (downhill or cross-country)	8
Jumping rope	11–12
Running (10 miles/16 kilometers per hour)	16

If your fitness level is less than 100% of your age-predicted fitness level, your first goal should be to become active. Your second goal should be to get as fit as possible and try to achieve your age-predicted fitness level for some duration of your workout. Remember, it's survival of the fittest. The more physically fit and active you are, the better your heart health and the longer and healthier your life will be.

Sex does not increase the chances for heart attack. Sex, in general, puts the same amount of pressure on your heart as a brisk 20-minute walk. As you get aroused your heart rate, breathing rate, and blood pressure elevate a little. During orgasm, the heart rate increases to anywhere between 90 beats per minute to 145 beats per minute. After orgasm your heart rate, breathing rate and blood pressure return to the resting levels. Only 1% of heart attacks are triggered by sexual activity (despite what television and movies would have you believe!).

Benefits of Physical Activity on the Heart

Running is the greatest metaphor for life, because you get out of it what you put into it.

— Oprah Winfrey

It is well established that if women are more physically active and physically fit, they will live longer and be less likely to die from a stroke or heart disease. Women who are physically active are less likely to develop cardiovascular disease, to say nothing of other diseases. So just how does physical activity reduce the risk of heart disease and stroke? Physical activity can help your heart in the following ways:

1. **Lower blood pressure**: Exercise can effectively lower blood pressure and should be part of the treatment for any high blood pressure diagnosis. Exercise can improve the arteries' ability to relax, allowing for better blood flow and improved ability of the arteries to respond to stress. A physically inactive woman has a 35% greater risk of developing high blood pressure, compared with women who are physically active.
2. **Boost metabolism:** Exercise increases calorie consumption; this can help with weight loss and weight maintenance.

3. **Prevent the development of diabetes:** The U.S.-based Diabetes Prevention Program (DPP) study showed that for an overweight person, combining an exercise program with diet changes reduced the risk of developing diabetes. Daily exercise appears to improve insulin production, which reduces the amount of sugar in the bloodstream.

4. **Improve diabetes control:** Regular physical activity can increase the body's insulin levels, helping to use blood sugar more effectively and improving blood sugar control. Exercise may even reverse the onset of diabetes.

5. **Improve cholesterol levels:** Regular activity can raise HDL (good) cholesterol and lower the LDL (bad) cholesterol (see Chapter 2). Even when an overweight person does not lose much weight with exercise, she can still use exercise to significantly improve her blood cholesterol levels.

6. **Improve circulation:** Exercise is one of few "prescriptions" that can reverse peripheral arterial disease and improve circulation where there is atherosclerosis in the peripheral arteries.

7. **Reduce stress, depression, and anxiety**: All three have adverse effects on the heart, and all can improve with regular physical activity. (See Chapter 10 for more about how stress affects heart health.)

8. **Lower the risk of a stroke:** Physical activity can lower the risk of a stroke, independent of its effects on lowering blood pressure and reducing cholesterol and the other beneficial effects of exercise on cardiac risk factors.

9. **Improve the function of the heart in heart failure patients:** Exercise, including resistance training, helps to build muscle. In addition, more and more research is showing that for people who suffer from heart failure, exercise can improve survival rates, symptoms, and quality of life. We highly encourage anyone with heart failure to discuss with their doctor if they can participate in a well-supervised exercise program, such as a cardiac rehabilitation program (see Chapter 6).

10. **Strengthen the heart muscle:** Remember that the heart is a muscle. The more you use it, the stronger it will be. Regular physical activity will improve your overall fitness because your heart muscle will be able to tolerate more exertion. Your resting heart rate will likely

reduce in response to regular exercise, too, because your heart won't need to work as hard to pump blood while you're at rest.

How Much Activity Do Women Need?

If your dog is fat, you're not getting enough exercise.

— Anonymous

With all the different exercise recommendations out there, knowing which to follow can be confusing. A friend's mother has been known to say, "I just meet the goal of the last guidelines, and then I am told to do more!"

Well, we want you to know that getting exercise doesn't have to be complicated, especially if you follow these five simple rules:

Rule #1: Just be active — doing something is better than doing nothing.
Rule #2: Make changes gradually, not abruptly, to avoid injury.
Rule #3: Before you start any exercise program, discuss with your doctor if it is safe to do so or if you need to have any testing done first.
Rule #4: Do activities you enjoy, whether you like dancing, gardening, or taking the dog for a walk. Have fun!
Rule #5: Remember that more is better. So move, move, move!

Various health agencies and fitness institutions have set similar guidelines for physical activity. Ultimately, they all aim to encourage women to move more. At one time, the recommendation was to exercise three days a week, it then changed to recommending exercising five days a week, but now it is recommended to exercise *most days of the week*, with five days a week being an absolute minimum. Women need to incorporate physical activity in their daily lives and make a concerted effort to increase the level or intensity of their workouts. If you do something every day, it will become a habit. Think of exercise like brushing your teeth: you wouldn't consider going a day without it.

Don't let what you cannot do interfere with what you can do.

—John Wooden

Guidelines and Recommendations for Physical Activity

American Heart Association Guidelines for Cardiovascular Disease Prevention in Women[4]	American College of Sports Medicine and American Heart Association Guidelines for Adults Under 65 Years[5]	American College of Sports Medicine and American Heart Association Guidelines for Adults Over the Age of 65 Years*[6]	Center for Disease Control[7]	Canada's Physical Activity Guide[8]
Do moderate-intensity activity, 60 minutes a day, most days of the week	Do moderate-intensity activity, 30 minutes a day, 5 days a week	Do moderate-intensity activity, 30 minutes a day, 5 days a week	Do moderate-intensity activity for 150 minutes of every week	Do endurance and flexibility exercises 4 to 7 days a week
	OR	OR	OR	
	Do vigorous-intensity activity, 20 minutes a day, 3 days a week	Do vigorous-intensity activity, 20 minutes a day, 3 days a week	Do vigorous-intensity activity for 75 minutes of every week	
	AND	AND	AND	AND
	Do 8–10 strength-training exercises, 8–12 repetitions of each exercise, 2 times per week	Do 8–10 strength-training exercises, 10–15 repetitions of each exercise, 2–3 times per week	Do muscle-strengthening activities 2 or more times per week	Do strength activities 2 to 4 days per week
		AND		AND
		If you are at risk of falling, perform balance exercises		Accumulate 60 minutes of physical activity every day to stay healthy or improve your health

*Also applies to adults 50 years and older with chronic disease conditions

Note: Moderate-intensity physical activity means exercise enough to raise your heart rate or break a sweat, while still being able to carry on a conversation (able to talk but not sing).

The basic theme one can take from all these recommendations is to exercise most days of the week, with the goal of raising your heart rate and breaking a sweat. We support the notion that some aerobic activity and muscle-stregthening exercises are needed on top of the routine activities of daily life. And all research agrees that more exercise is better. The minimum exercise of 30 minutes a day is for cardiac benefits. But for weight loss or weight maintenance, 60 to 90 minutes of activity a day is recommended. Given that two-thirds of our society is either overweight or obese, two-thirds of society needs to be moving more than the basic recommendations to lose weight and to reduce cardiovascular risk factors.

How to Become More Physically Active

There's no easy way out. If there were, I would have bought it. And believe me, it would be one of my favorite things!

— Oprah Winfrey

The hardest thing for most women is finding time to exercise. We all have many demands on our time — work, home, children, spouses, friends, parents . . . As women, we often give so much of ourselves that, when asked to list our priorities, we are the lowest on the list — if we're even on the list at all! But the fact is that you must take care of yourself in order to take care of others. Otherwise, you are of no use to anyone. Exercise will prolong your life and make you healthier if you remain active throughout your life. If you have never exercised, you will still benefit from starting to be physically active. It is never too late to get moving!

We know you lead a busy life, so the following sections give you some tips for how to *fit in fitness.*

Make an Appointment with Yourself
For women, the most important way to find time to be active is to schedule it in your calendar, just like all the other appointments you make (and keep). Designate and book this time just for you. You must make it, and yourself, a priority for that block of time in your day.

Just Move

It is important to just start moving. Do anything, because as we said in Rule #1, something is better than nothing, so do something every day. You really should have no day that doesn't include regular activity, even if it is just walking around your house, using the stairs, or walking to the post office — everything counts, except for sitting all day long. Always find a way to be active, even in the smallest ways. If you start looking for exercise in everything you do, you will be sure to find more ways to build it into your life.

Find 10 minutes

The benefits of exercise are cumulative. If you are just starting an exercise program, or if you are just too busy to find 30 minutes or an hour in your day when you can exercise, divide your workout into several 10-minute sessions. Research shows that moderate-intensity activity can be accumulated throughout the day in 10-minute bouts and is as effective as a longer, concentrated workout. And sometimes, if you are exercising only 10 minutes at a time, you can exercise more intensely than during one 30-minute workout.

We can all find 10 minutes in our day that we can spare for a bit of exercise. How about 10 minutes at the very beginning of your day, 10 minutes at lunchtime, and 10 minutes in the evening? A brisk walk, walking up the stairs at the office, running up and down the driveway a few times — these all count as your 10-minute sessions. If you can find 10 minutes to exercise three times a day, and you do this five times a week, you will have exercised 150 minutes in one week!

Mix It Up

Combine moderate and more intense workouts. Work out at a more comfortable pace, and then push it up a notch for either some part of your workout or on certain days. This is known as *interval training*. It will make your workouts more interesting, boost your metabolism, and help you lose weight. In addition, doing different workouts and different activities on different days may help you stick to exercise if you tend to get bored with the same routine. So mix it up!

Find a Friend

To help you start and stick with an exercise program, it can be helpful and fun to involve a friend or family member — he or she can help keep you motivated with your exercise plan and meeting your goals. Consider making it a family affair — making regular exercise a goal for your family sets a great example for your children, which will help them commit early to making regular activity a life-long habit.

Choose the Right Time

I have to exercise in the morning before my brain figures out what I'm doing.
— Marsha Doble

Choose the workout time that is best for you. For some people, it is morning. For others, it is late in the day. This may be because of your work schedule, your sleep habits, or how much flexibility you have in your day. Whichever time suits you best is the right time to exercise. Making it a habit to exercise during a specific time of day will make exercise, well, a habit.

Count It Out

Consider using a *pedometer* (a small device that counts the number of steps you take) to monitor your activity. This incredibly useful tool will provide you with feedback about just how active you are. A lot of women think they are very busy and active in their work because their feet hurt at the end of the day. But sometimes the real cause of foot pain is poor shoe choice! The reality is that most of our jobs are surprisingly sedentary. We sit an awful lot, more than we should be. A goal to "set" with your pedometer is 10,000 steps a day. If you walk 10,000 steps a day, you have walked 5 miles (8 kilometers), which is a lot more than what most people walk in a day. We recommend that you start by assessing the number of steps you take over a regular day. Then increase that number by about 500 steps a day for one week, then another 500 steps a day the next week, and so on, until you reach 10,000 steps a day. Sometimes, the value of seeing these numbers can be motivating and rewarding.

Be Creative

If you are on the lookout for ways to introduce activity into your daily life, you will find many ways to be active if you use a little creative thinking.

At home, doing housework and gardening is part of being active. If you are on the phone, don't sit — stand or walk instead. Make a rule not to drive to anywhere that is less than 1 mile (about 1.5 kilometers) from your house. (You will save gas and get exercise at the same time!) Walk the dog. And if you don't have a dog, offer to walk your neighbor's dog. If you must watch TV, place a bike or treadmill in front of it and use it whenever you're watching your favorite show. If you sit in front of the TV, get rid of your remote controls and get up when you want to change channels.

At work, walk to a person's office to relay a message instead of sending an email. Have meetings while walking. Stand if you are on a conference call. Take the stairs, rather than the elevator. Get off the subway or bus one stop earlier and walk a bit more to work every day. Use your lunchtime not only to eat but as a time to take a brisk walk. (Remember, even if you can find only 10 minutes to walk, do it!) Consider using an exercise ball as a chair at your desk to strengthen your abdominal muscles, improve your balance, and burn extra calories.

If you fly frequently for work or pleasure, walk in the airport to kill time if you are early for your flight. And when you travel, always pack your running shoes. Try to choose a hotel with a gym, and make sure you fit some workout time into your days.

Plan your weekend activities around physical activity. If you plan to go to the movies, walk there, or take a pre- or post-movie walk. If you must drive somewhere, park in the spot that is the farthest from the door — that's right, the one *farthest* away. You'll get exercise walking to the door.

If you start fitting fitness into your everyday life, you will soon stop thinking of it as a chore. Instead, you will find that fitting in more and more physical fitness is a satisfying challenge.

Exercise Your Options

If you get bored with your usual activities, try something new, like taking a class or joining a sports team. Many gyms offer trial memberships so you can try out their classes and equipment and see if you like them. Try yoga, Tai Chi, dance lessons, kickboxing, or any other activity that piques your interest. If you are new to exercise, consult with a personal trainer who can create a program tailored to your needs. Explore the options in your community. You may be surprised to find that your local community center may offer fitness programs that are free or cost much less than programs at mainstream gyms. And guess what? Video games that are interactive and keep you moving *do* count as exercise. Find any activity that you enjoy and do it. Exercise should be enjoyable, so find a way to make it fun so that you look forward to doing it.

The Heart of the Matter

Regular daily activity really is one of the most important things you can do for your heart. If you are not currently active, make the commitment today to take the first steps toward being active. Remember, every little bit counts. Many forms of exercise are free and can easily be integrated into even the busiest of schedules. Make exercise a priority in your life. Set aside time each day for exercise, just as you would for sleep or having breakfast. Whether it is taking a brisk walk, playing tennis, doing a fitness class, or participating in some other activity that you enjoy, aim to be active each and every day. Physical activity is key to saving your heart and improving your overall physical and emotional well-being.

Chapter 10

The Impact of Stress

Be master of your petty annoyances and conserve your energies
for the big, worthwhile things. It isn't the mountain ahead
that wears you out — it's the grain of sand in your shoe.
— Robert Service

Leslie is a single mother of two young children. She runs her own business, and in addition to taking care of her children, she is the primary caregiver for her elderly mother. Leslie works an average of 10 hours a day with her business, and on top of that, she shuttles the kids to and from school and to their after-school activities and does her best to squeeze in housework and visits to her mom's. Most nights she doesn't get to bed until almost midnight and is up at 6 a.m. preparing for the day ahead. Leslie says that she is stressed out all the time and she feels like her life is spinning out of control. She has no time for fun and friends, let alone exercise. She feels like she is being pulled in a million directions between her obligations with work, family, and managing the household. Leslie gets frequent colds, feels run-down and tired all the time, and has gained weight in the past few years. At her last doctor's appointment, she was told that her blood pressure and cholesterol are elevated and she is borderline diabetic. Her doctor warned her that unless she can lose weight and make some lifestyle adjustments, she will need medication.

You might know a woman like Leslie, or maybe you can relate to some aspects of her life and what she is going through. How often do you feel stressed out and struggle to cope with life's daily challenges? Stress has become a common and often debilitating force in our society. Many of us are living life in the fast lane — running from one commitment to the next with no time to relax, feeling pressed for time, anxious, overwhelmed, and basically stressed out.

Stress is the trash of modern life — we all generate it but if you don't dispose of it properly, it will pile up and overtake your life.

— Terri Guillemets

Our modern-day stress has become so constant that many of us do not even realize that it may be the underlying cause of our headaches, tight muscles, anxiety, racing heart, or difficulty sleeping. We think we are functioning okay and neglect these subtle symptoms. Yet, stress can have far-reaching effects on health. It can reduce immune function, impair libido and fertility, and cause weight gain. It is also an underlying factor in many serious chronic diseases, including heart disease, diabetes, and some cancers. It is estimated that 43% of all adults suffer adverse health effects from stress, and two-thirds of all visits to family physicians are due to stress-related symptoms.[1]

In this chapter, we'll talk about stress — what it is, how it affects your heart and the rest of your body, and what you can do about it. You will learn practical methods for managing stress through lifestyle modifications and relaxation techniques.

Understanding Stress

We often throw around the term "stress" in reference to how we feel when faced with unpleasant experiences, situations, or people, but what exactly does it mean? The first person to coin the term "stress" was Hans Selye, a Canadian endocrinologist. In 1936 he defined *stress* as "the non-specific response of the body to any demand for change." In other words, stress is how we respond internally to what is going on around us. In laboratory experiments, Dr. Selye discovered that animals subjected to physical and emotional stimuli (stress) such as blaring light, loud noise, or extreme temperatures all exhibited the same effects, namely stomach ulcerations, shrinkage of the thymus gland, and enlargement of the adrenal glands. In further experiments, Selye demonstrated that persistent stress could cause animals to develop diseases similar to those seen in humans — heart attacks, stroke, kidney disease, and rheumatoid arthritis. Selye's theories attracted worldwide attention, and stress soon became a buzzword.

> Stress can cause people to feel overwhelmed, anxious, and panicked. The American Psychological Association's 2007 Stress in America poll found that one-third of people in the United States report experiencing extreme levels of stress. In addition, nearly one in five report that they are experiencing high levels of stress 15 or more days per month.[2]

Good Stress, Bad Stress

Not all stress is bad for us. Some people find that they perform better or accomplish more when under stress. Low to moderate levels of occasional stress can be motivating and inspiring. It can push you to meet that looming deadline, help you to give an energetic presentation, or spur you to the finish line in a race.

But since most people tend to view stress as an unpleasant threat, Selye subsequently created a new word, *stressor*, to distinguish the stimulus from the response. Stress was the body's reaction or response to a situation or event, which is the stimulus or the stressor. Stress becomes harmful to our health when it is intense, chronic, and not managed properly. This is why stress has been referred to as "the spice of life or the kiss of death."[3] Stress can be positive or negative, depending on the context, how the event or situation is perceived, and how we react to it. Negative stress is sometimes referred to as *distress*.

The Stress Response

To understand why stress can be harmful to your health, it is important to look at what happens in your body when you are stressed. Think of how you might react in the following situation: *You are rushing to get to an important job interview. You are running late and a few blocks away from the interview you walk over a subway grate and break the heel of the favorite pair of shoes you're wearing.* You may feel stressed just picturing this scenario!

Your body undergoes a series of changes in what is called the stress response. There are three stages to this response: alarm, resistance, and exhaustion.

When the threat or stressor is identified or realized, the body responds in a state of *alarm*. Alarm is the startup stage, which defines the first reaction to the stressor. Stress hormones called *catecholamines* (adrenaline and noradrenaline) and *glucocorticoids* (cortisol) are released in the body. These hormones, which are secreted by the adrenal glands, prepare the body to fight; hence, this response is known as the *fight or flight response*. When this occurs, our body enters a catabolic state, where our fuels (glucose, fats, and amino acids) are broken down to provide energy. Heart rate, blood pressure, blood volume, and pulmonary (lung) tone increase to enhance the function of the heart and lungs. Muscle tone increases to improve strength and performance. *The fear and pressure is likely evident on your face.*

The second stage is *resistance*. If the stressor persists *(and in this case it does)*, it becomes necessary to attempt some means of coping with the stress. Although the body begins to try to adapt to the strains or demands of the environment, the body cannot keep this up indefinitely, so its resources are gradually depleted. *You broke your heel, you don't have another pair of shoes with you, a lot is riding on this job interview, and you are already late. You frantically try to reattach the heel, but it doesn't work. So, heel in hand, you start running to make it to the interview. Now you are worried about how you are going to look arriving at the interview late, flustered, and with a broken heel.*

The third and final stage is exhaustion. The body's resources are depleted and the body is unable to maintain normal function. *Your heart is racing and you are visibly perspiring. You feel frustrated and can't think straight. You are on the verge of tears as you try to pull it together.*

This stress response, an innate mechanism, was designed to help us cope with short bursts of stress, such as running from a predator. The problem is that our bodies have not adapted to handle a continuous onslaught of stress, and the continuous release of stress hormones.

Are You Stressed Out?

We all react differently to our stressors. Some of us seem to handle them better than others. There are those who seem cool as cucumbers and don't let anything get to them, while others overreact to the slightest thing. But there are also people who, on the outside, seem to handle stress well, but inside they worry and suffer the effects of stress, such as anxiety and sleeplessness.

How we respond to stress depends on our personality type, our coping skills, and how we are conditioned from a young age to deal with stressful life situations. There is some commonality though among the underlying causes or sources of stress. According to the Stress in America poll, work, money, children and family issues, health concerns, housing costs, and intimate relationships are the leading sources of stress today.[4] We are sure we could all add a few other sources to that list, too.

To check your stress level, take a few minutes to complete this Stress Index:

Do you frequently . . .	Yes	No
Neglect your diet?		
Try to do everything yourself?		
"Blow up" easily?		
Seek unrealistic goals?		
Fail to see the humor in situations others find funny?		
Act rudely?		
Make a "big deal" out of everything?		
Look to other people to make things happen?		
Have difficulty making decisions?		
Complain you are disorganized?		
Avoid people whose ideas are different from your own?		
Keep everything inside?		
Neglect exercise?		
Have few supportive relationships?		
Use sleeping pills and tranquilizers without a doctor's approval?		
Get too little rest?		
Get angry when you are kept waiting?		
Ignore stress symptoms?		
Put things off until later?		
Think there is only one right way to do something?		

Do you frequently . . .	Yes	No
Fail to build relaxation time into your day?		
Gossip?		
Race through your day?		
Spend a lot of time complaining about the past?		
Fail to get a break from the noise and the crowds?		
Score 1 for each Yes answer, 0 for each No answer	Total Score	

What does your score mean?

1 to 6: There are few hassles in your life, but you don't avoid problems by shying away from challenges.

7 to 13: You are in fairly good control of your life. Work on the choices and habits that may be causing unnecessary stress.

14 to 20: You are approaching the danger zone. You may be experiencing stress-related symptoms and strain in your relationships. Think carefully about the choices you make and take time to relax every day.

Above 20: Emergency! You must take time now to work on your attitude, make changes to your diet, exercise, and relax.

"Stress Index" reproduced with permission from The Canadian Mental Health Association, Ottawa, Ontario

Women and Stress: Our Changing Roles

To understand why stress has become such a serious issue, particularly for women today, it is important to look at how the lives of women in the Western world have changed over the past several decades. Until the modern industrialized times, women focused on taking care of their spouses, children, and households. We did not play a significant role in the workforce — social, cultural, and religious practices, and lack of access to education had limited our ability to do so. Would you believe that many universities did not even offer degrees for women until the 1940s?

At the end of the nineteenth century, a U.S. census report revealed that women made up only 15% of the total workforce. This started to change in the twentieth century with World War I, as the demands on the production sector rose and women began to occupy more jobs in factories. As occupations evolved and women gained access to higher education, we started to play a stronger role in other areas of the workforce.

Does stress affect women more than men?

According to a U.S. survey examining the effects of stress and its impact on our lives, women experience more stress than men, report more physical symptoms of stress than men, and are also more likely than men to think they manage their stress poorly.[5] This survey also reported the following:

♥ Women more commonly report experiencing extreme stress than men and are more concerned with stress.

♥ Women react to stress differently from men and are more likely to exhibit a physical symptom of stress.

♥ Women are more likely to report consequences of stress, such as sleep problems, overeating, skipping meals, and using prescription medications.

♥ Twenty-four percent of women with sleep problems report a loss of more than an hour of sleep nightly.

In 1950 in the United States, about one in three women participated in the labor force. By 1998, nearly three of every five women of working age were in the labor force. As of 2009 in the United States, women held 49.83% of the nation's 132 million jobs.[6] And in Canada as of 2006, women accounted for 47% of the workforce.[7] This is a dramatic shift from just a generation ago that has changed how we women spend our days. Our responsibilities have grown dramatically, which has had a significant impact on many areas of our lives, including our levels of stress.

Today, in addition to having careers, women frequently have primary responsibility for home and family matters — providing the majority of care to children, spouses, parents, parents-in-law, friends, and neighbors. And we also play many other roles: hands-on health provider, care manager, friend, companion, surrogate decision-maker, and advocate.[8]

Marital stress worsens the prognosis in women with heart disease.

Many studies have looked at the role of women and family caregiving. Consider the following:

♥ It is estimated that from 59 to 75% of family or informal caregivers are women.[9]

♥ Although men also provide assistance, women still shoulder the major burden of care. Some studies show female caregivers may spend as much as 50% more time providing care than male caregivers.[10]

In our efforts to take care of everyone, often it is ourselves who suffer. Several studies have found that higher levels of stress, depression, anxiety, and other mental health challenges are common among women who care for an older relative or friend. Giving so much to others can have a substantial impact on our own health.

Stress and Your Health

It is well known that our emotional state can affect our physical or biological state. Many studies have found that people who are positive, optimistic, and don't worry excessively (don't sweat the small stuff) have less chronic disease and live longer.

Stress has the very opposite effect on health. It literally wreaks havoc on almost every system in the body. The most commonly experienced consequences are headaches, insomnia, anxiety, stiff muscles, and upset stomach. Stress also hampers immune function, memory, and concentration; impairs fertility and reduces sex drive; and can accelerate the aging process. Stress is linked to some of our most serious and debilitating diseases, namely heart disease, diabetes, and cancer.

Not feeling stressed?

Absence of symptoms does not mean the absence of stress. You may not exhibit the common and obvious symptoms of stress, but stress could still be impacting your health. Likewise, camouflaging symptoms of stress with tranquilizers or relaxant drugs may deprive you of the signals that tell you to reduce the strain on your body.

Stress and Heart Disease

The mind-body connection is particularly meaningful when it comes to the health of your heart. Studies that have compared the effects of various psychosocial factors on cardiac-related outcomes generally suggest that when stress persists over time, even seemingly low levels can be toxic, particularly among those with established disease.[11]

Researchers have identified five negative psychological states that, to varying extents, increase cardiovascular disease risk: hopelessness, pessimism, rumination, anxiety, and anger/hostility.[12] (*Rumination* in this sense refers to the tendency to think repetitively and passively, often about situations that caused negative emotions, and to focus on these symptoms of distress.)

In one large international study called the INTERHEART study, over 90% of patients with heart attack had one or more of nine major cardiovascular risk factors, and psychosocial stress was among the leading risk factors.[13] In men, research has found that high levels of hostility predict heart disease more often than other common risk factors such as high cholesterol, cigarette smoking, or obesity.[14]

Dr. Hilary Tindle and colleagues studied the effect of *optimism* (positive future expectations) versus cynical, hostile attitudes toward others in relation to heart disease specifically in women. In their study, 97,253 women from the Women's Health Initiative who were free of cancer and cardiovascular disease when they entered the study were assessed over an eight-year period. They found that *optimists had lower rates of heart disease and total mortality* and that the most cynical, hostile women had higher rates of heart disease and total mortality.[15] This points to the significant impact that attitude and outlook have on our risk of heart disease and even death. Later in this chapter we discuss how you can shift your thinking and become more positive and optimistic.

Stress can also impact other risk factors for heart disease, such as:

♥ *Blood pressure:* Stress hormones (adrenaline) increase your blood pressure by causing your heart to beat faster and your blood vessels to narrow. Short-term increases in blood pressure due to stress are not a problem, but when this occurs continuously it can cause damage to your blood vessels and heart.

♥ *Cholesterol:* Stress hormones (adrenaline and cortisol) trigger the production of cholesterol to provide the body with energy and repair damaged cells. Cortisol has the additional effect of creating more sugar (the body's short-term energy source). In recurrent stressful situations, sugars are repeatedly unused and are eventually converted into triglycerides or other fatty acids. Research also suggests that these fatty deposits are more likely to end up in the abdomen, and those with more abdominal fat (a pot belly) are at higher risk for cardiovascular disease and diabetes.

♥ *Blood clots:* The surge in adrenaline caused by intense stress causes the blood to clot more easily, increasing the risk of heart attack and stroke.

♥ *Inflammation:* Inflammation appears to be associated with the development of atherosclerosis, the process in which fatty deposits build up in the inner lining of arteries. Several studies have shown that chronic stress can lead to a chronic inflammatory process that is implicated in heart disease.[16]

Burnout

Inflammation can be measured by looking at levels of fibrinogen and C-reactive protein. In one particular study, researchers looked at the impact of burnout in working men and women. Burnout symptoms were measured by a questionnaire that asked participants to rate their level of fatigue, cognitive weariness (poor concentration), and emotional exhaustion. In women, symptoms of burnout were associated with higher levels of C-reactive protein and fibrinogen concentrations, reflecting higher levels of inflammation in those women with more symptoms of burnout.[17]

♥ *Lifestyle factors:* Stress can trigger people to engage in behaviors that are harmful to the heart, including smoking, drinking, overeating, and eating unhealthy or comfort foods such as sugary, salty, or high-fat snacks.

Does Stress Affect Women's Hearts Differently than Men's?

We know that women react and handle stress differently than men, but is there also a difference in how stress affects a woman's heart compared to a man's? The answer is, quite possibly, yes. A growing body of research suggests that stress can have a more profound effect on women's hearts.

In one study looking at job stress, researchers found that the predictive power of psychosocial risk factors, including burnout, on future *cardiovascular events* (heart attack or stroke) was higher among women than among men.[18] A study released in 2010, involving over 17,000 women, found that women who reported high job stress faced a 40% increase in heart disease, compared to women with less job stress. Women who worried about losing their jobs were more likely to be overweight or to have higher blood pressure and cholesterol, all risk factors for heart disease.[19]

Another issue related to stress that seems to affect women more than men is the *Broken Heart Syndrome*. This syndrome can occur after hearing shocking news that results in sudden emotional stress. There is an acute surge in adrenalin and other stress hormones that can temporarily "stun" the heart, resulting in heart muscle weakness and symptoms that appear just like a heart attack. The good news is that most people show dramatic improvement of the heart muscle function within a few days and complete recovery by two weeks, based on the best study of this syndrome from Johns Hopkins University researchers. In this study of 19 patients, 18 of whom were women, the emotional events that triggered this syndrome were news of a death, shock from a surprise party, a fear of public speaking, armed robbery, a court appearance, and a car accident. A hallmark feature of the syndrome was the heart's unique contraction pattern, as viewed by an ultrasound (echocardiogram) of the heart: the bottom of the left ventricle contracted normally, but the middle and upper portions of the left ventricle were weakened.[20]

Strategies for Surviving Stress

We can't avoid stress; it really is an inevitable part of life. Nor is there a quick-fix approach for managing stress. Although medications such as sedatives may be prescribed, we feel that these drugs should be reserved for severe cases that do not respond to lifestyle approaches. These medications cause serious side effects and can lead to addiction.

A successful program for managing stress involves a holistic approach: learning strategies and tools to cope with stress, getting regular exercise, and following a healthful diet. There are also some supplements, discussed below, that can help support the body during stress and promote relaxation.

Managing Stress

There are countless stress-management books and programs available, and though some are helpful, many can be a bit overwhelming, requiring drastic lifestyle changes that are not always possible. Here we outline a practical four-step plan, with suggestions on how to identify and manage stress and create more balance in your life.

1. Identify Your Stressors

This first step in managing stress is to identify the sources of your stress — your *stressors* or *triggers*. These are the thoughts or events that make you feel stressed, or the people who push your buttons. To do this, it is helpful to keep a journal or notepad handy so that when you feel stressed you can make a note of the circumstances. Whether it is situations at work or home, with family or friends, make a note of how you felt, how you reacted, and how you coped. Are your current coping strategies helpful, or do they make matters worse? Identifying your stressors and making notes of how you deal with stressful situations will help you in creating a stress-management plan.

2. Adopt Stress-Management Strategies

There are many positive ways to deal with stress. Since we all have different triggers and different ways of responding to and coping with stress, you will need to experiment with the various techniques and strategies outlined below. Keep in mind that you may need to adopt several of these strategies to help deal with your stressors. Adopt those that make you feel calm and in control. Try one or two to start, gradually incorporating as many as you can into your life:

♥ **Avoid negative people and people who stress you out.** We're talking about the chronic complainers, those who never have anything nice to say, and those who seem to enjoy criticizing. If being around someone consistently makes you feel stressed, limit the amount of time you spend with that person or end the relationship entirely.

♥ **Avoid the things that cause you the most stress.** You might also find ways to alter stressful situations so that they are more tolerable. For example, if traffic is a trigger, see if you can change your work hours to minimize driving in rush hour or take a different route, even if it is longer. If that is not possible, try listening to music, news, or an audio book while driving to make the time more enjoyable.

♥ **Train your mind to react differently to current triggers.** Look at life's challenges as opportunities. This may take some time and practice. You will need to really examine how you think and react in various situations and come up with ways to change your reactions. For example, if you find it stressful giving a speech, look at it as an opportunity to develop your public-speaking skills. You can take a course or work with a coach. With practice, you will find public speaking less stressful.

♥ **Develop a positive attitude.** Positive thinking lessens stress, makes you feel happy, and makes others want to be around you. Start off by being positive each day. List things you like about yourself, your achievements, your family, or your plans for the day; when you're feeling stressed, take time to reflect on all the positive things in your life. No matter how bad a situation may seem, try to find a bright side or positive aspect to focus on.

♥ **Work on managing anger and hostility.** This takes time. Practice controlling or redirecting your frustrations into a positive action. If you have had a bad day at work, rather than get into a fight with your partner or children, go for a walk or a bike ride. This will help relieve the stress and put your energy into something more positive.

If you are patient in one moment of anger, you will escape a hundred days of sorrow.

— Anonymous

♥ **Take charge.** Express your feelings and be assertive. This will make you feel more in control and less like a victim of circumstances. Deal with problems up front; ignoring them or keeping them inside can lead to anger, resentment, helplessness, and anxiety. Work on communicating your thoughts and feelings with friends, family, or a counselor.

♥ **Look at the big picture.** Sometimes we get caught up stressing over the small stuff. When you're faced with something that causes you stress, ask yourself if it is really that important, whether it will matter in a week or month, and if it is worth getting upset over. If the answers are no, let your worries and negative thoughts go and redirect your energy to things that matter.

♥ **Let go of perfectionism.** Having high standards for yourself and others can set you up for unnecessary stress. Instead, set reasonable standards or expectations, and realize that perfection is not always achievable or necessary.

♥ **Learn to compromise.** When in a dispute, finding some common ground or meeting a person halfway can leave both of you feeling more satisfied.

3. Create Balance

For fast-acting relief, try slowing down.

— Lily Tomlin

For many women, working too much and not having time to relax and enjoy family and friends are common sources of stress and can lead to burnout, frustration, anxiety, and sleeplessness. It is important to create balance in your life, take time for yourself, and enjoy social activities. Here are some suggestions to achieve this:

♥ Schedule time for yourself each day, even if it is only a half hour. Set aside time to recharge your batteries and do something you enjoy, such as exercising, gardening, talking with friends, or taking a bath.

♥ Learn to say no. Taking on more than you can handle and being overextended, either with work or other commitments, can lead to stress. Know your limits. Set boundaries and stick to them. This can be challenging but also liberating. Just try it and see how you feel.

♥ Work on improving your time-management skills. Running late for appointments, squeezing too much into your day, and multitasking can be stressful. If your schedule is getting out of control, prioritize your activities and work on accomplishing only the most important items. Leave the extras for another day or cut them out completely. Delegating responsibilities is another helpful time-management strategy. If you find large projects overwhelming, try breaking them down into smaller projects.

I try to take one day at a time, but sometimes several days attack me at once.

— Jennifer Yane

4. Accept the Things You Can't Change

Some sources of stress are unavoidable or beyond our control, such as dealing with a serious illness, losing a loved one, or living in hard economic times. These are events that you cannot change. In these cases, it is essential to accept the situation and move forward. Dwelling on the negative leads to stress, frustration, and feelings of helplessness. Keep these points in mind:

♥ Rather than feeling stressed over things you cannot change, try to focus on the things that are in your control, such as your own thoughts, behaviors, and actions.

♥ Look for the positives in a situation. Even during tough times, you can find opportunities to learn and experience personal growth. Try reframing the problem and looking at it in a different light.

♥ Learn to forgive. Holding a grudge or feeling angry and resentful leads to stress and negative emotions. While it is not always easy, work on forgiving and accepting.

♥ Maintain a sense of humor. Being able to laugh at yourself when you make a mistake and finding the humor and levity in challenging situations are great ways to relieve stress.

> *Laughing relaxes and expands blood vessels, which helps protect the heart.*

Food and Mood

Your dietary choices have a significant impact on your emotional well-being and your ability to cope with stress. A healthy diet provides your body with sustained energy and the nutrients it needs to recuperate, regenerate, and repair.

In Chapter 8 we discussed our nutritional recommendations for a healthy heart. Those same foods will also help support your body in dealing with stress. As well, keep the following nutritional points in mind:

♥ Start your day right, with breakfast — it really is the most important meal of the day. It will set the tone for how you feel, both physically and emotionally. Without breakfast you may have low blood sugar and fatigue, which can impair how you handle stress. Try oatmeal with cinnamon and flaxseed, yogurt and berries, or poached eggs with whole-grain toast. These foods provide quality sources of protein and carbohydrates, which will help support proper blood sugar levels and give you sustained energy.

♥ Eat small, frequent meals throughout the day. This will keep you energized and in a better position to deal with stress. In fact, it is much better to eat five small meals a day than three larger meals.

♥ Choose low-glycemic carbohydrates such as whole-wheat pasta, whole-grain breads, brown rice, fruits, and vegetables. These foods contain essential nutrients to help the body deal with stress and promote better blood sugar levels, which in turn is helpful to your emotional well-being.

♥ Ensure you eat enough protein. Protein provides sustained energy and is required for muscle repair and growth. Choose lean poultry, fish, beans, legumes, nuts, and seeds.

♥ Drink lots of purified water and calming herbal teas, including chamomile, lemon balm, and passionflower.

♥ Eat more fish, flaxseed, hemp, and chia seed. These foods contain essential fatty acids that your brain and nervous system need.

Certain foods and drinks can worsen your response to stress, make you anxious and irritable, and prevent you from sleeping well. Aim to minimize or avoid these foods:

♥ Caffeine, common in coffee and soft drinks, can trigger and worsen stress. Ironically, many people turn to these drinks when feeling stressed or tired, yet they can actually increase the secretion of adrenaline and cortisol, making you more edgy and stressed. Plus, the temporary boost of energy is often followed by fatigue, which leaves you feeling even worse. If you are currently consuming a lot of caffeinated beverages (three or more cups daily), wean yourself off them slowly to avoid withdrawal symptoms. Caffeine withdrawal can be quite severe, causing irritability, depression, muscle pain, headaches, and anxiety. Try switching your morning coffee or soda to green tea. Green tea has much less caffeine and contains an amino acid called L-theanine that promotes calming and relaxation.

♥ Alcohol, which is commonly thought of as a relaxant, can actually worsen the effects of stress. Alcohol is a diuretic, meaning it causes the body to lose water. The body senses dehydration as a stressor, and, as a result, cortisol levels rise. Alcohol can also impair sleep. One drink may make you feel drowsy and help you fall asleep; several drinks can increase nighttime awakenings and impair restorative sleep. Limit alcohol to one to two drinks per day.

♥ Sugary foods cause fluctuations in blood sugar, which may cause mood swings and worsen the effects of stress. Cut down on candy, baked goods, sweet condiments (e.g., ketchup), and snack foods.

♥ Fast food and processed foods (snack foods) are high in saturated fat and sugar, and low in nutrients. These foods can also trigger anxiety and mood swings.

Supplements for Stress

There is no product, drug, or supplement that can make your stress go away. Stress is how you respond to what is going on around you. However, some supplements help mitigate the effects of stress and can be helpful, for example, by promoting relaxation and calmness, reducing cortisol and stress hormones, improving sleep, and generally supporting the body's needs during times of stress.

B vitamins

The B-complex vitamins are known as "stress vitamins" because of the vital role they play in the health of the nervous system and adrenal function. They also act as coenzymes in many of the body's metabolic reactions. Niacin (vitamin B3) is required to metabolize *tryptophan*, and tryptophan is a precursor to *serotonin*, a neurotransmitter that calms the mind. Vitamins B6 and B12 are necessary for the nervous system to work properly. Vitamin B5 (*pantothenic acid*) plays an important role in stress relief. Stress can deplete B vitamins, and a deficiency of these vitamins can actually cause anxiety and worsen the body's response to stress. You can get your B vitamins as part of a multivitamin or take a B-complex separately. Look for a product that provides 50 to 100 mg of the B vitamins. Multivitamins are discussed in more detail in Chapter 7.

L-theanine

Over the past few decades, countless studies have revealed that the antioxidants in green tea benefit heart health, cancer prevention, weight loss, digestion, cognitive function, immune function, and more. But there is another component of green tea that is gaining popularity: *L-theanine*. An amino acid that occurs naturally in tea plants, L-theanine is found in the highest concentration in green tea leaves. It creates green tea's characteristic *umami* or "fifth taste" (besides the four traditional tastes of sweet, sour, salty, and bitter), sometimes described as savory.

L-theanine supplements

L-theanine offers a wide range of benefits for stress management: it promotes calm and relaxation, improves sleep quality, and heightens mental clarity and focus. The most studied form of L-theanine is Suntheanine, and it is widely available in supplements, along with some healthy beverages, like Vitamin Water B-Relaxed. The recommended dosage of Suntheanine is 50 to 200 mg. It can be taken daily or as needed during times of stress. Suntheanine's effects are generally felt within 30 minutes and have been shown to last 8 to 12 hours. Unlike prescription tranquilizers, Suntheanine does not cause any serious side effects — no drowsiness or addiction.

Adaptogens

Several herbs are said to have adaptogenic properties. An *adaptogen* helps the body adapt to stresses of various kinds, whether heat, cold, exertion, trauma, sleep deprivation, or psychological stress. One herb that is widely touted as an adaptogen is *Panax ginseng*. Some research suggests that Panax ginseng can help support physical and mental performance, immune function, and adrenal gland function, all of which can be hampered by stress.

Another adaptogen is *ashwagandha*, an Ayurvedic herb. Sensoril, a patented form of the herb ashwagandha, has been shown to help increase the body's resistance to stress, fatigue, and tension, and to boost energy levels. In one clinical study, Sensoril was shown to significantly reduce stress symptoms, including fatigue, flushing, sweating, palpitations, sleeplessness, irritability, and the inability to concentrate. The study also found that supplementing with Sensoril significantly reduced cortisol levels and increased dehydroepiandrosterone (DHEA) — both of these hormones are adversely affected by stress. And there were side benefits, too — Sensoril reduced fasting blood sugar and improved lipid levels (meaning it had a positive effect on LDL and HDL cholesterol and triglycerides).[21]

Milk's calming effect

It has long been known that babies are calmer and even sleepy after drinking milk. And how many of us have been told to have a glass of warm milk before bed? There is actually some science to support the calming properties of milk. In recent years, researchers have discovered a peptide (protein compound) that is present in milk and has relaxing properties. Preliminary research conducted on a supplement called Lactium that contains this peptide shows it can help reduce the physical and mental effects and symptoms of stress.

It is not necessary to take all of these supplements. They each work differently and offer various benefits. Review your options and talk to your healthcare practitioner for guidance in choosing the right products for you.

Are women being over-medicated?

Drugs that are often prescribed for stress, especially when it occurs with depression or anxiety, are the selective serotonin reuptake inhibitors (SSRIs), which include fluoxetine (Prozac), sertraline (Zoloft), fluvoxamine (Luvox), paroxetine (Paxil), and citalopram (Celexa). Since women are more likely to see their doctors when feeling stressed, anxious, or depressed, and also more likely to talk about their feelings, it is not surprising that they are more medicated than men. In fact, according to a report issued by the U.S.-based National Center for Health Statistics, more than twice as many antidepressants are prescribed for women as for men, and more than one in three doctor's office visits by women involved a prescription for an antidepressant.[22] These drugs are associated with numerous side effects, including sleep disturbances, weight gain, and sexual dysfunction. And in some cases, antidepressants can worsen stress and anxiety.

The time to relax is when you don't have time for it.

— Sydney J. Harris

Relaxation Techniques

As discussed in Chapter 9, exercise is incredibly beneficial for your heart and is also a great stress reliever. In fact, the benefits of exercise in relieving stress are more powerful than any prescription drug. When we exercise, there is a release of hormones called *endorphins* into the bloodstream. These hormones boost our mood, relieve stress, and improve our overall sense of well-being. Exercise improves blood flow to the brain, bringing with it additional sugars and oxygen that may be needed in times of mental strain. Increased blood flow to the muscles can help relax tense and sore muscles. Exercise also improves sleep quality, and getting a good night's sleep is critical for coping with stress.

· In addition to getting regular exercise, consider these specific techniques to help take the edge off stress:

Yoga

Yoga has been practiced for centuries by many cultures around the world. It is now recognized to be an effective method for reducing stress, improving flexibility and strength, and improving sleep and overall health. Some studies have shown that yoga can help lower blood pressure.

The word *yoga* means "union" in Sanskrit, the language of ancient India where yoga originated. Yoga is the union occurring between the mind, body, and spirit. Yoga is about creating balance in the body through developing strength and flexibility. This is accomplished by performing poses or postures, each of which has specific physical benefits. The poses can be done quickly in succession, creating heat in the body through movement, or more slowly to increase stamina and perfect the posture of the pose. There are several traditions or types of yoga, each with its own approach, though all with the same goal.

Yoga is suitable for people of all ages. The best way to learn yoga is to join a class. Yoga DVDs may be helpful, but to learn proper technique, we recommend taking a class led by a qualified instructor. Once you learn the basics, yoga is something that you can practice on a mat in the comfort of your own home.

Massage

Stress can cause tension to build up in the muscles, causing a decrease in circulation and nutrient delivery to tissues that results in "knots" or sore muscles. These knots can be painful, inhibit your ability to perform daily tasks, and even impair sleep quality. Massage — whether it be Swedish massage, Shiatsu, aromatherapy massage, Thai massage, or sports massage — can help by increasing blood flow to the muscles and tissues, which helps loosen stiff, sore muscles; promotes relaxation; increases the removal of metabolic waste; and promotes nutrient delivery to healing tissue. Massage can also boost your immune system, which may be compromised by chronic stress.

Acupuncture

A treatment in traditional Chinese medicine, *acupuncture* is based on the philosophy that living beings have a vital energy, called *qi*, that circulates through 12 invisible energy lines on the body known as *meridians*. Each meridian is associated with a different organ system. It is thought that an imbalance in the flow of qi throughout a meridian leads to disease and health problems.

According to Chinese medicine, stress, anxiety, depression, or any strong emotion interrupts the smooth flow of energy throughout the body. This can lead to pain, muscle tension, and other health problems. To restore balance to the flow of energy, an acupuncturist inserts fine needles into specified points along meridian lines. There are more than 1000 acupuncture points on the body.

Western medicine has gradually come to accept and even endorse the benefits of acupuncture. It is thought that acupuncture helps alleviate stress by releasing endorphins — the brain's natural pain-killing chemicals. Acupuncture also improves blood circulation, which oxygenates the tissues and cycles out cortisol and other waste chemicals. The calming nature of acupuncture also decreases heart rate, lowers blood pressure, and relaxes the muscles.

Deep Breathing

Sometimes the most important thing in a whole day is the rest we take between two deep breaths.

— Etty Hillesum

When you are feeling stressed, it is a common reaction to hold your breath or take short shallow breaths from the chest rather than the abdomen. This can reduce oxygenation, lower energy levels, and worsen the effects of stress.

Deep breathing, also known as belly breathing or diaphragmatic breathing, is a simple yet effective technique to reduce stress. This type of breathing increases oxygen levels in the body and has a calming effect.

Deep breathing can be done anytime and anywhere. To practice this technique, sit comfortably in a quiet area. Take a deep breath in through your nose, counting from one to four as you breathe in. Exhale through your mouth as you count down from four to one. Repeat 20 or 30 times. Try to practice deep breathing several times throughout the day, especially when you are feeling stressed.

Qigong

Qigong (pronounced "chee-gong") is a series of ancient Chinese exercises that use breathing and visualization to improve mental, physical, and spiritual health. Qigong can help reduce stress and improve sleep. A review of nine clinical studies involving over 900 people found that self-practiced qigong for less than one year was effective in decreasing blood pressure in patients with essential hypertension (high blood pressure with no identifiable cause).[23]

Visualization

Visualization, also known as mental imagery, is a method of connecting mind and body to promote relaxation and healing. It allows us to escape our stressful reality for a brief time and focus on thoughts that are calming and relaxing. To practice visualization, simply sit or lie down in a quiet, comfortable spot and close your eyes. Visualize a scene or place that makes you feel calm and happy. It could be a memory from childhood or a pleasurable vacation. Focus on the sights and sounds of this scene and imagine that you are there. Relax and enjoy.

Meditation

Meditation is a mental discipline that has been practiced for more than 5,000 years among Eastern cultures. It is a component of almost all religions. Today, it is commonly practiced in the West, outside of religion, for stress management. Meditation involves turning attention to a single point of reference and entering into a deep state of relaxation. There are numerous meditative disciplines involving a wide range of spiritual and/or psychophysical practices. They emphasize different goals, including achieving a higher state of consciousness, greater focus, creativity, self-awareness, or simply a more relaxed and peaceful frame of mind.

Aside from promoting calmness, relaxation, and a sense of peace, meditation offers a number of other benefits: it slows heart rate and breathing, normalizes blood pressure, improves oxygenation, and reduces sweating. Meditation can lower cortisol levels, improve immune system function, and slow the aging process. It also helps clear the mind and boost creativity. Meditation has even been used to help people overcome addictions to alcohol, cigarettes, and drugs.

To meditate, go to a quiet area and sit in a comfortable chair or cross-legged on the floor. Close your eyes and work on clearing your head. You may focus on a sound, like *om,* or on your own breathing, or on nothing at all. Try to hush the inner voices and thoughts so that you can achieve internal silence. This is not easy to do, especially if you lead a busy life and are feeling stressed. It will take some practice, but eventually you will be able to let go of your thoughts and enjoy the feeling of relaxation. Allow yourself 10 to 20 minutes to meditate.

Meditation is something you can do anytime and anywhere. Again, it takes some practice, but the time and effort are worthwhile. Meditation is incredibly effective for reducing stress and improving emotional and physical well-being. The effects can be felt in just one session, but it also offers long-lasting benefits. If you need guidance, consult with an instructor.

There is more to life than increasing its speed.
— Mohandas K. Gandhi

The Heart of the Matter

Stress is an inevitable part of our lives — we can't avoid it, so finding effective coping strategies is essential for maintaining physical and emotional health. Not only will your heart benefit, but you will find that you sleep better at night, think more clearly during the day, and have an overall better sense of well-being. Fortunately, adopting these strategies is not as difficult as you might think.

Chapter 11
Sleep and Heart Health

The bed is a bundle of paradoxes: we go to it with reluctance, yet we quit it with regret; we make up our minds every night to leave it early, but we make up our bodies every morning to keep it late.
— Charles Caleb Colton

Sleep is one of our body's most vital needs. Just like air, food, and water, it is essential for life. It is often thought of as a passive state, yet during sleep our body's major organs and regulatory systems are busy repairing, restoring, and regenerating themselves. Sleep is required for the rejuvenation of our immune, nervous, skeletal, and muscular systems, and various hormones are secreted during sleep. Just like stress, lack of sleep is associated with many health problems, including an increased risk of heart disease. Considering the hectic pace of life today, it is not surprising that sleep deprivation has become a common concern, especially for women.

Sleep is also one of the first things to be sacrificed when we are busy. Just think of how often you cut your sleep time short so that you can fit more into your day. We try to get by with five or six hours of sleep, but the reality is that sleep deprivation, particularly when chronic, takes its toll on our health. And let us clear up a common misconception: you can't go without sleep during the week and catch up on the weekend. There is no sleep bank, and there is no way to catch up on lost sleep.

In this chapter we explain why sleep is so important for your heart and overall health, tell you about what factors affect sleep, and suggest strategies to improve the quality of your sleep.

The stress-sleep connection

Lack of sleep often goes hand in hand with stress. When we are worried, anxious, and stressed we often have difficulty sleeping at night, and a lack of sleep can make us more reactive to the stressors we face. Just think of how you feel when you don't get a good night's sleep. The next day you are tired and more easily irritated and stressed.

Are We Sleep Deprived?

Sleep deprivation has become a major issue, particularly for women. A number of surveys have reported that women are more likely than men to have difficulty falling and staying asleep and to experience more daytime sleepiness. According to a recent Sleep in America poll conducted by the U.S. National Sleep Foundation, more than half of American women (60%) say they get a good night's sleep only a few nights per week or less, and 67% say they frequently experience a sleep problem. The majority of women (80%) reported having trouble sleeping because of worrying too much and/or being stressed out or anxious (79%). According to 43% of survey participants, daytime sleepiness interferes with their daily activities, and poor quality of sleep affects virtually every aspect of their time-pressed lives — they report being late for work, stressed out, too tired for sex, and having little time for their friends.[1]

Not only are we having difficulty sleeping, but we are sleeping less. In 1998, only 12% of people reported getting less than six hours of sleep on weeknights. In 2009, that figure rose to 20%.[2] This is likely a reflection of our increasingly busy schedules and lack of time for sleep. Although our society has changed, our brains and bodies have not. We have simply not adapted to be able to handle sleep deprivation and, as a result, our health is suffering.

People who say they sleep like a baby usually don't have one.

— Leo J. Burke

Sleep Disorders

Here are the most common types of sleep disorders that affect women:

♥ *Insomnia:* Difficulty falling asleep or staying asleep, waking up too early, and feeling tired. Insomnia is more common among women than it is among men. It is often caused by stress, depression, anxiety, or as a side effect of medication.

♥ *Obstructive sleep apnea:* A condition in which a person's airway narrows or totally collapses during sleep, causing a temporary pause in breathing. It often happens several times throughout the night, so the person's quality of sleep is poor. It is estimated that sleep apnea affects about 2% of women, but after middle-age, 9% of women are affected.

♥ *Snoring:* During sleep, breathing causes the tissue at the back of your throat to vibrate and make noise. It can awaken both the snorer and her partner.

♥ *Restless legs syndrome:* A condition characterized by an intense urge to move your legs in response to uncomfortable or odd sensations. This urge gets stronger at night when you are trying to sleep and is relieved only by moving your legs. Restless legs syndrome affects nearly twice as many women as it does men.

♥ *Nightmares:* Bad dreams can cause you to wake from sleep. Nightmares affect women more often than men. Not only do they disturb sleep, but they can even cause a fear of sleep.

Most people do not consider dawn to be an attractive experience — unless they are still up.

— Ellen Goodman

Sleep Deprivation and Your Health

A lack of sleep is associated with a host of health problems, including the following:

♥ Memory loss and poor concentration.
♥ Irritability, anxiety, and mood swings.

♥ Depression. There is a reciprocal relationship between the two: sleep problems may cause or contribute to depressive disorders and depression can cause difficulty sleeping.

♥ Weight gain. Lack of sleep can impact hormones that regulate appetite and metabolism.

♥ Reduced immune function. Sleep deprivation alters immune function, including the activity of the body's killer cells, and can increase the risk of infection and illness.

♥ Diabetes. People who get less than six hours of sleep each night have a higher risk of developing pre-diabetes, a condition that precedes the diagnosis of diabetes and is characterized by impaired fasting glucose and insulin resistance.

♥ Accelerated aging. Sleep deprivation stresses the body and triggers the release of stress hormones that promote inflammation. Lack of sleep also lowers levels of *human growth hormone* (HGH), and low levels of HGH are associated with gaining of body fat, loss of lean muscle tissue, brittle bones, and thin, wrinkle-prone skin.

♥ Heart attack and stroke. Lack of sleep increases risk factors for heart attack and stroke. (The next section discusses this risk in more detail.)

♥ Cancer. Some studies have shown that lack of sleep (six hours or less at night) significantly increases the risk of breast cancer.

Is a lack of sleep making you fat?

Recent research has found a connection between lack of sleep and weight gain. Lack of sleep can increase levels of a hormone called ghrelin, which increases appetite. Levels of another hormone called leptin, which helps signal when we are full, are lowered when we are sleep deprived. Metabolism is also lowered when you go without adequate sleep. Plus, the feelings of fatigue and hunger are similar and can be confused — we tend to eat when we're actually sleepy because we think fatigue is a sign of hunger.

Sleep and Heart Disease

Sleep deprivation can increase our risk of heart disease in several ways: it increases blood pressure, triggers inflammation, promotes calcium buildup in the arteries (which leads to plaque formation), and may cause an irregular heartbeat.

Physicians call early morning "the witching hour" for heart attacks because most heart attacks occur in the morning, when stress hormones, such as cortisol, peak. Additionally, blood is thicker and harder to pump because a person is partially dehydrated.

The exact way in which lack of sleep causes these problems is still being explored. Researchers speculate that sleep deprivation puts the body into a state of high alert, increasing the production of stress hormones. This raises blood pressure and cortisol levels (promoting inflammation), which are major risk factors for heart attack and stroke. Some research has found that sleep influences the functioning of the lining inside blood vessels. Sleep allows the heart to slow down and blood pressure to drop for a significant part of the 24-hour day. If a person is sleeping less, there are shorter periods of lower blood pressure, and this can increase the risk of plaque being dislodged from the blood vessels, which can rupture and cause a heart attack or stroke.

Studies also show that sleep apnea increases the risk of stroke. When a person stops breathing, the lack of oxygen elicits the fight or flight response (see Chapter 10), which increases adrenalin production. This causes blood pressure to rise and the blood to clot more easily, increasing the risk of stroke.

Signs of heart attack in women

Research indicates that women often experience new or different physical symptoms as long as a month or more before experiencing heart attacks. The symptoms most commonly reported by women are unusual fatigue (70.6%), sleep disturbance (47.8%), and shortness of breath (42.1%). Surprisingly, 43% of women in this study reported having no chest pain during any phase of the attack.[3]

The Breaking Point
Experts agree that we should be striving for seven to eight hours of sleep at night. But at what point does our lack of sleep impact our hearts? That has been the subject of several recent studies.

In one large study, researchers looked at 71,617 female health professionals (aged 45 to 65) without reported coronary heart disease at baseline, who were enrolled in the Nurses' Health Study. They wanted to determine if an association exists between decreased sleep duration and an increased risk of coronary events such as heart attack. Participants were followed for 10 years. Researchers found that shorter daily sleep duration (in participants who got six hours or less) was associated with an increased risk of heart disease, independent of other risk factors such as smoking and higher body mass.[4]

In 2007, a study published in the medical journal *Hypertension* suggested that women who routinely sleep fewer than seven hours a night may have an increased risk of developing high blood pressure. The study followed 10,300 adults between the ages of 35 and 55 for five years. When compared with women who typically slept seven hours each night, women who slept six hours a night were 42% more likely to develop high blood pressure. Women who routinely slept no more than five hours had a 31% higher risk. In contrast, this study did not show a relationship between sleep deprivation and high blood pressure in men.[5]

Another study by researchers at the University of Chicago found that lack of sleep promoted calcium buildup in the heart arteries, leading to plaques that can then break apart and cause heart attacks and strokes. They evaluated 495 men and women aged 35 to 47 and found that 27% of those who got less than five hours of sleep each night showed plaque in their heart vessels (a symptom of atherosclerosis), whereas only 6% of subjects who slept more than seven hours each night showed such plaque buildup. They also determined that getting a mere one hour less sleep on average each night can increase coronary calcium by 16% — coronary artery calcification is a predictor of coronary heart disease.[6]

A study published in the journal *Sleep* found that women who get less than five hours' sleep per night had elevated levels of high sensitivity C-reactive protein (hs-CRP) in their blood. As discussed in Chapter 2, hs-CRP is a marker of inflammation and elevated levels are associated with risk of heart disease. Interestingly, lack of sleep did not cause the same rise in hs-CRP in men.[7]

The breaking point for lack of sleep and stroke risk also appears to be in the same range. One recent study found that postmenopausal women who regularly sleep less than six hours or more than nine hours a night may have an increased risk of ischemic stroke. Researchers looked at sleep duration in a group of 93,175 older women (aged 50 to 79) in the Women's Health Initiative Observational study. Their aim was to examine the women's risk of ischemic stroke in relation to the number of hours they reported sleeping. The study found that women who reported sleeping six hours or less were at 14% greater risk of stroke than those who slept seven hours a night. And, surprisingly, women who reported sleeping for longer periods (greater than nine hours) were actually at greater risk. In this study, the risk of ischemic stroke was 60 to 70% higher for those who slept nine hours or more. The authors concluded that habitual sleep patterns are important in determining postmenopausal women's risk of ischemic stroke, and the underlying adverse effect of long sleep requires further study.[8]

The best cure for insomnia is a Monday morning.

— Author unknown

Sleep Hygiene

As we've shown, sleep is essential for good health; a lack of sleep can increase your risk of heart disease and other health problems. Getting a good night's sleep also puts you in a better position to deal with the stresses of the day ahead. So to improve your quality of sleep, work on developing good sleep hygiene habits. Consider these tips for getting a better night's rest:

- ♥ *Set aside at least seven to eight hours for sleep.* Leaving only five or six hours for sleep may make you feel stressed and make it harder to fall asleep.
- ♥ *Get into the habit of going bed and waking up at the same time every day,* such as 10 p.m. for sleep and 6 a.m. to wake.
- ♥ *Do relaxing activities before bed.* For example, read a book, take a warm bath, or meditate.
- ♥ *Reserve your bedroom for intimacy and sleep only;* don't work or watch television in your bedroom.
- ♥ *Make your bedroom dark, quiet, and comfortable.* Create an environment that is calming and relaxing. Use room-darkening shades or heavy curtains to keep the light out. This will help trigger your body's release of *melatonin,* a hormone that helps us fall asleep and regenerates cells. If you live in a loud neighborhood, try using a fan to create white noise, which will help mask the sounds around you.

♥ *Avoid long naps during the day.* If you are really tired during the day and need a nap, limit it to 30 to 45 minutes. Anything longer than that can affect your sleep at night.

♥ *Exercise regularly, but not before bed.* Exercise is stimulating; exercising too close to bedtime can make it difficult to fall asleep.

♥ *Avoid caffeine* (coffee, tea, soda, and chocolate) six hours before bedtime. Caffeine is stimulating and can affect sleep quality.

♥ *Avoid alcohol within four to six hours of bedtime.* Alcohol may help you fall asleep, but as the alcohol levels in your blood start to fall, it can have a stimulant effect, causing you to wake up in the night. So limit alcohol in the evening or avoid it completely.

♥ *Choose your bedtime snacks wisely.* Sugary foods, like cookies, ice cream, and candy bars, can cause a "sugar rush" and keep you from falling asleep. Avoid these foods within four hours of bedtime. Also avoid heavy and spicy foods before bed, as they can trigger heartburn and acid reflux and affect your ability to stay asleep. If you want a bedtime snack, choose a food that contains *tryptophan*, an amino acid that stimulates the release of *serotonin*, a brain chemical that facilitates sleep. Examples of good bedtime snacks include whole-grain crackers and cheese, turkey, a banana, or a small bowl of cereal.

♥ *Be aware that some medications can contribute to sleep problems.* Among them are antihistamines and decongestants, beta blockers, thyroid medications, antidepressants, and pain medications (containing caffeine).

Prescription Drugs for Insomnia

The main class of drugs used for treating insomnia and sleep disorders are the *benzodiazepines*, namely alprazolam (Xanax), clonazepam (Rivotril), diazepam (Valium), and lorazepam (Ativan). These sedative/tranquilizer drugs work quickly (within 30 to 60 minutes) to ease anxiety and promote relaxation and sleep; however, they can cause side effects such as loss of coordination, dizziness, and memory impairment. And, ironically, over time these drugs can actually impair sleep quality.

Benzodiazepines are highly addictive. Some people can develop a tolerance, so they will need a higher dosage to get the same effect. Unfortunately, many people suffer with the consequences of relying on prescription sedatives. When they are taken for an extended period (more than two weeks), they become habit-forming. Stopping these medications can cause horrible withdrawal symptoms — heightened anxiety, confusion, memory loss, and even seizures.

Natural Remedies for Sleep

Many natural products are promoted to help with sleep. Some of these have been researched, whereas others are considered in the realm of folklore or tradition. Options to consider include:

♥ *Valerian* — an herb with sedative properties. It may be helpful for managing chronic sleep disorders, anxiety, and restlessness. Valerian is a little slower to work and is usually well tolerated, but it may cause some next-day drowsiness. Valerian should not be combined with prescription sleep aids. The dosage varies depending on the concentration of active ingredient and *formulation* (tablet or tincture), so check with a healthcare practitioner before taking this product.

♥ *Melatonin* — a hormone secreted from the pineal gland in the brain that regulates our sleep-wake cycles. Supplements of synthetic melatonin have been studied and found to be helpful for improving sleep quality, especially in people who work night shifts or travel to different time zones. Melatonin does not cause next-day drowsiness. It has been suggested that melatonin can interfere with blood clotting and potentially increase the effects of anti-coagulant drugs. The typical dosage is 3 to 6 mg one hour before bedtime.

Other natural products that are promoted to help with sleep include chamomile, passionflower, and skullcap; however, there is no reliable scientific evidence that these remedies work.

The Heart of the Matter

Now that you know the value of sleep and how a lack of sleep can increase your risk of heart disease and other health problems, it is obvious that you need to make sleep a priority. So, the next time you are tempted to cut short your sleep time to squeeze in more work or take care of the needs of others, keep this in mind: you can never make up for lost sleep time, and as much as those around you may appreciate your extra work and efforts, they also want you to be alive and healthy in the future.

Aim for the recommended seven to eight hours a night, and if you are having a hard time sleeping, review our list of sleep hygiene tips (earlier in this chapter) and determine if any of your lifestyle habits are interfering with your sleep.

Chapter 12

Why Women Matter:
Marching to a New Beat

I don't mind living in a man's world, as long as I can be a woman in it.

— Marilyn Monroe

If you recall from the Introduction, heart disease is the number-one killer of women. Worldwide, one out of every three women will die from heart disease. In comparison, one out of every 30 women will die from breast cancer. In fact, in the United States, more women than men have died from heart disease and stroke since 1985.[1] What is truly amazing is that, still, almost one in two women does not recognize that heart disease is the leading cause of death among women and does not recognize this as a health issue of concern.[2] Many women don't even know that if they experience chest pain or have other symptoms of heart disease, they should call 9-1-1. Are you shocked? Amazed? Does it make you ask why, as women, we are better informed about breast cancer, and the need to screen for that disease, than we are about our number-one killer? This is a good question to ask, but it does not have an easy answer.

Heartfelt Research

Until the turn of the twenty-first century, the medical community did not know much about the risk of heart disease in women. Research done on heart disease was predominately done on men, and very few studies included women. And this continued, despite the fact that more women were dying of heart disease than men, and indeed, there was a notable decline in deaths from heart disease among men, as more aggressive and life-saving treatments became available. It appeared that although treatments were improving, women were less likely to have these treatment offered to them, and if they were offered, it was often too late to make a difference in women's outcomes.

In 1991, the first female director of the National Institutes of Health (NIH) was appointed. This woman, a cardiologist named Dr. Bernadine Healy, was a champion of women and heart disease who would lead the charge to get needed research on women and their hearts. She established a policy whereby the NIH could fund only clinical trials that included *both* men and women if the condition being studied affected both sexes. She also directed $625 million from the NIH to study the effect of hormone replacement therapy on heart disease in women in the landmark trial known as the Women's Health Initiative. This important study began in the 1990s and would go on to reveal that hormone replacement therapy was, in fact, not beneficial in reducing the risk of developing heart disease. These findings changed the care of millions of women around the world in a dramatic way. But the 1990s was not that long ago, and the results from such studies are only emerging in this last decade. Hence, we are just starting to understand women's hearts and to see where the gender differences exist. And since women currently comprise less than a quarter of all heart-related research, we still have a lot of work to do.

Gender Differences

What we do know is that women, compared with men, have worse outcomes if they are diagnosed with heart disease or undergo heart-related procedures. Women are more likely to die from a heart attack than men, particularly younger women. Women under the age of 50 who have a heart attack are twice as likely to die from it, compared with men under the age of 50. Women are still less aggressively treated after having symptoms of angina.[3] They are less likely to undergo testing that is usually done for symptomatic heart disease and less likely to get necessary medications. Ultimately, this results in women having poorly controlled symptoms, an increased risk of a heart attack, and in more women dying from their heart disease over time. When we look at the statistics from hospitals across the United States in women who have had a heart attack, we continue to see this increased risk for women, particularly among African American women. Women are more likely than men to die in hospital after a heart attack, with African American women being at the highest risk.[4] Women are less likely to get the proven life-saving medications after the heart attack or upon discharge from the hospital,[5] they (particularly African American women) are less likely to get the interventions (like angioplasty, stent, thrombolytics and coronary artery bypass surgery) that can improve blood flow after a heart attack, and they are also more likely to have bleeding complications after treatment of a heart attack, resulting in both a longer hospital stay and higher death rates.[6]

Similarly, when a woman undergoes coronary bypass surgery, her outcomes are worse than a man's, and this has been the case for almost 30 years. Women have almost twice the chance of dying during surgery than men. Of course, women tend to be older when they undergo surgery; they often have other diseases, like diabetes, hypertension, or other vascular diseases. And surgery is more often an emergency procedure in women, rather than being an elective procedure, compared with men. Nonetheless, women are less likely to be smokers and usually have less damage to their hearts than men. They also usually have fewer diseased coronary arteries. But as with heart attacks, the younger a woman is, the greater her risk of dying in the hospital after coronary bypass surgery — the reason for this is unclear.[7] If women survive the surgery, they have a more difficult time recovering from it, even if their pre-surgery health status is taken into account.[8] But there is good news about coronary bypass surgery in women. Recent analysis of outcomes after coronary bypass surgery in British Columbia have shown that the operative mortality has decreased for both men and women, and it appears that the number of patients who died within 30 days of their coronary bypass surgery is equal (approximately 2%) for both men and women, although there was still a higher mortality rate in women under the age of 50, compared with men of that age.[9] Another favorable study for women is related to coronary bypass surgery when it is done without stopping the heart, a procedure known as *off-pump* bypass surgery. Based on statistics recorded in the large Society of Thoracic Surgeons (STS) National database, women and men seem to do equally well when off-pump coronary bypass surgery is performed. However, this surgery is technically more challenging than conventional bypass surgery and so it is done only for certain people.[10]

There are many other gender differences in outcomes and treatment of heart disease. We know that pacemakers and implantable cardioverter defibrillators (ICDs) are used less often in women than in men, in both Canada and the United States, despite women meeting the criteria for implantation.[11] There is some debate about whether women benefit as much as men from these devices, but we should not be withholding potentially life-saving treatment from women while we wait for this answer. High blood pressure is more common in women than men after the age of 65, yet treatment to get blood pressure controlled is poorer in women than in men, putting women at a greater risk for a heart attack or stroke. Women with high cholesterol are less likely than men to have their LDL cholesterol at their target level compared, particularly if they are diabetic.[12]

It is because of these gender differences that we want to empower all women to be aware of what we know and don't know right now about women and their hearts. We want you to be able to discuss your cardiac risk factors, treatment goals, medication choices, and therapies with your doctor. If you are aware of the life-saving properties or the risk-reducing goals, you can be more involved with your treatment plan and ask the right questions if treatments are not offered. Sometimes, a certain treatment may not be an option for certain people, but if that is the case for you, then you deserve to know why. We are women and we are women at risk for heart disease, so we want every woman (including ourselves) to be offered the best treatment available to reduce the risk of heart disease and improve our survival as a group. Just because we are not like men and may not exhibit the same symptoms as men, we still deserve excellent care for our hearts. After all, do we really have to change the foot just because the shoe doesn't fit? Or do we just need to find the perfect shoe that does fit?

It takes a really big man to fill my shoes.

— Madonna

What We Know about Our Hearts

At the beginning of the book we asked you to fill out a survey to test your knowledge about heart health. This survey was conducted among a group of 135 women in Pompano Beach, Florida. Why don't you go ahead and take it again now? You may be surprised by how much you have learned about your heart and heart disease and about what you need to do on the path to heart health. (Indeed, we bet you will know all the answers!) After you have taken the test again, take a moment to refer back to your earlier answers to see just how far you've come. We'll discuss the answers below.

Pompano Beach Heart Survey

1. What is your number-one health concern?
    A. Breast cancer
    B. Cervical cancer
    C. Lung disease
    D. Heart disease
    E. Mental illness
    F. Other

2. What is the number-one killer of women?
    A. Breast cancer
    B. Cervical cancer
    C. Lung cancer
    D. Heart disease
    E. Suicide

3. Have you ever been screened for heart disease?
    A. Yes
    B. No

4. Do you think you are at risk for heart disease?
    A. Yes
    B. No

5. What is the lifetime risk of heart disease?
    A. One in three women will develop heart disease in their lifetime.
    B. One in 100 women will develop heart disease in their lifetime.

C. One in 1000 women will develop heart disease in their lifetime.
D. One in 10,000 women will develop heart disease in their lifetime.

6. Which supplement is recommended for heart disease prevention?
    A. Folic acid
    B. Vitamin E
    C. Vitamin C
    D. Fish oil (omega-3)
    E. Beta-carotene

7. What is normal blood pressure?
    A. Less than 100/70
    B. Less than 120/80
    C. Less than 135/85
    D. Less than 140/90

8. What is normal body mass index (BMI)?
    A. Less than 25 kg/m^2
    B. Less than 30 kg/m^2
    C. Less than 35 kg/m^2
    D. I am unaware of what the body mass index is.

9. Which supplement should all women take daily to prevent heart disease?
    A. Aspirin (81 mg)
    B. Aspirin (325 mg)
    C. Folate
    D. None of the above
    E. All of the above

10. Which of the following are risk factors for heart disease in women?
    A. Tobacco use
    B. Physical inactivity
    C. Family history of heart disease
    D. All of the above
    E. None of the above

11. At what age should women be screened for heart disease
    A. Age 60 and above
    B. Age 50 and above
    C. Age 40 and above
    D. Age 30 and above
    E. Age 20 and above

12. After a woman under the age of 60 has a heart attack, she is more likely to survive compared to a man of the same age who has a heart attack.
    A. Yes
    B. No

13. Does hormone replacement therapy protect women against heart disease?
    A. Yes
    B. No

14. How informed about heart disease do you feel you are?
    A. Poorly informed
    B. Moderately informed
    C. Highly informed

The women in our sample area were an average age of 46 years old (but ranged from ages 19 to 94), with 59% being white, 29% African American, 10% Hispanic, and the remainder Asian, South-Asian, or any other race/ethnicity.

We were happy to find that the majority of our survey respondants knew that the number-one killer of women was heart disease, so we were surprised that the number-one health concern for these women was breast cancer, with 33% reporting this. However, heart disease was a close second, with 24% reporting heart disease as being their major health concern. The majority (60%) of the women in this survery had not been screened for heart disease, and most women (63%) did not believe that they were at risk for the disease. Only 44% correctly responded that the lifetime risk of heart disease was one in three. Almost two-thirds of the women knew that fish oil (containing omega-3s) is recommended for heart disease prevention over other supplements. Only 7% of women knew that a "normal" blood pressure is less than 120/80 mmHg, with the majority (73%) believing that normal blood pressure was less than 135/85 mmHg. The majority of women did not know what the body mass index (BMI) was, but the majority of those who did know what BMI was were aware that a normal BMI is less than 25 kg/m^2. Fifty-five percent of this sample thought that all women should take 81 mg of aspirin daily, but this was sort of a trick question, because the answer really depends on age. Almost all women were aware that all the risk factors we listed were risk factors for heart disease, since 81% correctly answered question 10. Most of our survey responders thought that you should be screened for heart disease at or after the age of 40, when in fact we recommend that screening for heart disease begin at age 20 — only 4% got this answer correct. Almost half of the surveyed women seemed aware that for a young woman (under the age of 60) who has a heart attack, her *odds of survival are lower* than a similar-aged man who has a heart attack (so the answer here would be "No"). We were greatly surprised to find that 53% of women still thought that hormone replacement therapy may protect women against heart disease, although, admittedly, 35% of women did not answer this question. We speculate that this represented the fact that there is a lot of confusion about this matter and women did not know the answer, since the remainder of the questions were all answered and not left blank. Only 6% of our surveyed women felt that they were highly informed about heart disease, which is when we realized the need for this book.

If we are not highly informed about heart disease, if we don't how to protect ourselves, or what screening we require, or what medications or supplements are beneficial (or harmful), it is hard for us to protect ourselves and reduce our risk of developing the disease. Heart disease *is* preventable, but it is only recently that women and their hearts have started to be studied. It is also only recently that guidelines specific to women have been established. And it is only recently that we as doctors have been reaching out to women to help them be informed about their number-one killer. So it is understandable that women still need more information on heart disease prevention, because the cardiology community is still in the infancy of its campaign to really educate women. This kind of thing doesn't happen overnight. Our goal is to help women become informed about their risk of heart disease and learn how to reduce that risk.

Working to Save Our Hearts

You put high heels on and you change.

— Manolo Blahnik

As women, we need to work to save our hearts. If we don't start doing it, who will? It is never too early and absolutely never too late to make changes that can improve cardiac risk factors, improve heart health, and give you a better chance of living free from cardiovascular disease. Even if you already have cardiovascular disease, making changes toward a more heart-healthy lifestyle can mean the difference between a healthier life, free of further heart disease or strokes, versus one that's not.

Making changes can be overwhelming, but it is possible. We advise you to start with small steps. What are the easiest things for you to change? Do those first. Set small goals and work toward them. Then set another goal, then another, and another . . . You get the point: baby steps. The truth is, for most people, overly dramatic changes rarely stick in the long term. And we want any changes you make to stick with you for a lifetime. So whether you need to lower the salt in your diet, or reduce the fat in your foods, or start exercising — or all three — you will succeed if you have a plan for how to make the changes gradually, how they will fit into your life, and how you can monitor the effect of any change you make.

Change is rarely easy, but it is always possible. Discussing your plan and goals with your doctor or other healthcare provider will help you stay on track and monitor your progress. Sometimes it takes a while to see the effects of change. The one many of our patients struggle with is related to weight loss, because it can be hard to see the weight change, despite making adjustments in diet and increasing activity. But it is not just about weight — the weight will come off eventually — often, other factors start changing first: muscle mass increases, metabolism increases, beneficial changes to cholesterol and blood pressure occur. Keeping track of all facets of your progress and seeing your physician regularly can give you positive reinforcement that your body is responding to your hard work.

Faith is taking the first step, even when you don't see the whole staircase.

— Martin Luther King, Jr.

Sometimes you have to have faith, but when you cannot see the effect of your changes, it also helps to have some science to back you up.

Advocacy, Education, and Knowledge

We really are just beginning to understand what is going on in women's hearts, and change goes beyond the measures that we take to improve our individual heart health. What we need and deserve is further research in the area of heart disease prevention and treatment in women. We need to continue, as a community, to push for our governments to support this research. And given that women are still underrepresented in the heart research published to date, we need to push our politicians and leaders to understand how this disease impacts women and just how many women it has the power to affect. We need to figure out why our patterns of heart disease appear to be different from men's. We need to determine how to recognize symptoms and detect heart disease earlier in women. We need to understand why women seem to have more bleeding risks related to our treatments and determine if these can be prevented. We still need to understand why women seem relatively protected from heart disease until menopause, yet hormone replacement therapy does not improve cardiac outcomes. We need to study women of different races to understand how race can affect cardiac risk factors and the heart. We need to determine the impact of our changing society on our future cardiovascular risk: we are getting heavier as a nation, we eat more calorie-dense foods, and diabetes is on the rise. Heart disease may increase in this younger generation as a consequence, and we may see a change in our population — where the older generation outlives the younger generation for the first time.

We also need educational programs and guidelines to help doctors understand women's unique issues and keep up to date on emerging research. And we need current educational programs for women to continue, so women understand what puts their hearts at risk and what they can do to reduce their risk. We also need public policy that targets preventive strategies to improve heart health and reduce stroke in women. We need to create public and health policy that will reward preventive screening for heart disease in women. Our health policy currently encourages mammograms to screen for breast cancer, yet breast cancer is not nearly as deadly as heart disease. Breast cancer is often curable, yet women who are diagnosed with heart disease live with it for the rest of their lives. We need to create a "cardiac mammogram" of sorts, a standard screening for heart disease that is routinely done on women and covered by any type of health coverage. Lastly, we need women to feel empowered to enroll in clinical trials of heart disease and heart disease prevention because, ultimately, without research on women, we cannot find the answers that will benefit current and future generations.

The Heart of the Matter

To end with some words of wisdom, we can't say it any better than Ms. Oprah Winfrey:

> *My philosophy is that not only are you responsible for your life, but doing the best at this moment puts you in the best place for the next moment.*

By taking responsibility for our lives, and by encouraging our public officials to increase research on women and our number-one killer, we can all be empowered to improve our health and, ultimately, save our hearts.

Endnotes

Introduction

1. Lloyd-Jones D, et al. "Heart Disease and Stroke Statistics — 2009 Update: A Report from the American Heart Association Statistics Committee and Stroke Statistics Subcommittee." *Circulation* (2009), 119(3):480–486.

2. Mosca L, et al. "Twelve-Year Follow-Up of American Women's Awareness of Cardiovascular Disease Risk and Barriers to Heart Health." *Circulation: Cardiovascular Quality and Outcomes* (2010), 3(2):120–127.

3. Rosamond W, et al. "Heart Disease and Stroke Statistics —2007 Update: A Report from the American Heart Association Statistics Committee and Stroke Statistics Subcommittee." *Circulation* (2007), 115(5):e69–171.

4. Wenger, NK. "You've Come a Long Way, Baby. Cardiovascular Health and Disease in Women: Problems and Prospects." *Circulation* (2004), 109(5):558–560.

5. See #3.

Chapter 2

1. Sabanayagam C and Shankar A. "Sleep Duration and Cardiovascular Disease: Results from the National Health Interview Survey." *Sleep* (2010), 33(8):1037–1042.

2. Ridker P, Danielson E, Fonseca F, et al. "Rosuvastatin to Prevent Vascular Events in Men and Women with Elevated C-Reactive Protein." *The New England Journal of Medicine* (2008), 359(21):2195–2207.

3. Brunzell JD, Davidson M, Furberg CD, Goldberg RB, Howard BV, Stein JH, Witztum JL. "Lipoprotein Management in Patients with Cardiometabolic Risk: Consensus Conference Report from the American Diabetes Association and the American College of Cardiology Foundation." *Journal of American College of Cardiology* (2008), 51(15):1512-1524.

Chapter 3

1. Mosca L, Banka CL, Benjamin EJ, Berra K, Bushnell C, Ganiats T, Gomes AS, Gornick H, Gracia C, Gulati M, Haan CK, Judelson RD, Keenan N, Kelepouris E, Michos E, Oparil S, Ouyang P, Oz M, Petitti D, Pinn VW, Redberg R, Scott R, Sherif K, Smith S, Sopko G, Steinhorn RH, Stone NJ, Taubert K, Todd BA, Urbina E, Wenger N. "American Heart Association Evidence-Based Guidelines for Cardiovascular Disease Prevention in Women." *Circulation* (2007), 115(11):1481–1501.

2. Lloyd-Jones DM, Leip EP, Larson MG, D'Agostino RB, Beiser A, Wilson PW, Wolf PA, Levy D. "Prediction of Lifetime Risk for Cardiovascular Disease by Risk Factor Burden at 50 Years of Age." *Circulation* (2006), 113(6):791–798.

3. Lloyd-Jones, DM. "Cardiovascular Risk Prediction: Basic Concepts, Current Status, and Future Directions." *Circulation* (2010), 121(15):1768–1777.

Chapter 4

1. Raman, Subha, et al. "Real-Time Cine and Myocardial Perfusion with Treadmill Exercise Stress Cardiovascular Magnetic Resonance in Patients Referred for Stress SPECT." *Journal of Cardiovascular Magnetic Resonance* (2010), 12:41.

2. Expert Panel on the Detection, Evaluation, and Treatment of High Blood Cholesterol in Adults: Executive summary of the Third Report of the National Cholesterol Education Program (NCEP) Expert Panel on the Detection, Evaluation, and Treatment of High Blood Cholesterol in Adults (Adult Treatment Panel III). *Journal of the American Medical Association* (2001), 285(19):2486–2497.

Chapter 6

1. "Randomized Trial of Cholesterol Lowering in 4444 Patients with Coronary Heart disease: The Scandinavian Simvastatin Survival Study (4S)." *The Lancet* (1994), 344(8934):1383–1389.

2. Sacks FM, Pfeffer MA, Moye LA, et al. "The Effect of Pravastatin on Coronary Events after Myocardial Infarction in Patients with Average Cholesterol Levels. Cholesterol and Recurrent Events Trial Investigators." *The New England Journal of Medicine* (1996), 335(14):1001–1009.

3. "Prevention of Cardiovascular Events and Death with Pravastatin Patients with Coronary Heart Disease and a Broad Range of Initial Cholesterol Level. The Long-Term Intervention with Pravastatin in Ischemic Disease (LIPID) Study Group." *The New England Journal of Medicine* (1998), 339(19):1349–1357.

4. GISSI-Prevenzione Investigators. "Dietary Supplementation with N-3 Polyunsaturated Fatty Acids and Vitamin E after Myocardial Infarction: Results of the GISSI-Prevenzione Trial." *The Lancet* (1999), 354(9177):447–455.

5. GISSI-HF Investigators. "Effect of N-3 Polyunsaturated Fatty Acids in Patients with Chronic Heart Failure (The GISSI-HF Trial): A Randomised, Double-Blind, Placebo-Controlled Trial." *The Lancet* (2008), 372(9645):1223–1230.

6. "Expert Panel on the Detection, Evaluation, and Treatment of High Blood Cholesterol in Adults: Executive Summary of the Third Report of the National Cholesterol Education Program (NCEP) Expert Panel on the Detection, Evaluation, and Treatment of High Blood Cholesterol in Adults (Adult Treatment Panel III)." *The Journal of the American Medical Association* (2001), 285(19):2486–2497.

Chapter 7

1. *Nutrition Business Journal*. "NBJ Reviews the $25 Billion U.S. Supplement Market." Accessed April 3, 2010. http://nutritionbusinessjournal.com/pressreleases/NBJ-reviews-US-Supplement-Market/

2. *National Center for Complementary and Alternative Medicine*. "Using Dietary Supplements Wisely." http://nccam.nih.gov/health/supplements/wiseuse.htm and Health Canada. "Baseline Natural Health Products Survey Among Consumers, March 2005." Accessed April 5, 2010. http://www.hc-sc.gc.ca/dhp-mps/prodnatur/index-eng.php

3. *U.S. Food and Drug Administration*. "Overview of Dietary Supplements." Accessed April 6, 2010. http://www.fda.gov/Food/DietarySupplements/ConsumerInformation/ucm110417.htm#what

4.   *Health Canada.* "Natural Health Products." Accessed April 6, 2010. http://www.hc-sc.gc.ca/dhp-mps/prodnatur/index-eng.php

5.   Worthington V, Nutritional Value of Organic versus Conventional Fruits, Vegetables and Grains. *The Journal of Alternative and Complementary Medicine* (2001), 7(2):161–173.

6.   Wang C, Chung M, Lichtenstein A, et al. "Effects of Omega-3 Fatty Acids on Cardiovascular Disease." Evidence Report/Technology Assessment No. 94. AHRQ Publication No. 04-E009-2. Rockville, MD: *Agency for Healthcare Research and Quality* (March 2004).

7.   Mosca L, Banka CL, Benjamin EJ, et al. "Evidence-Based Guidelines for Cardiovascular Disease Prevention in Women: 2007 Update." *Circulation* (2007), 115(11):1481–1501.

8.   *Medline Plus.* "Niacin." Accessed April 13, 2010. http://www.nlm.nih.gov/medlineplus/druginfo/natural/patient-niacin.html

9.   Gordon RY, Cooperman T, Obermeyer W, et al. "Marked Variability of Monacolin Levels in Commercial Red Yeast Rice Products: Buyer Beware!" *Archives of Internal Medicine* 2010, 170(19):1722–1727.

10.   Schurks M, Glynn RJ, Rist PM, et al. "Effects of Vitamin E on Stroke Subtypes: Meta-Analysis of Randomised Controlled Trials." *British Medical Journal* 2010, 341:c5702.

Chapter 8

1.   Jakobsen MU, Dethlefsen C, Joensen AM, et al. "Intake of Carbohydrates Compared with Intake of Saturated Fatty Acids and Risk of Myocardial Infarction: Importance of the Glycemic Index." *The American Journal of Clinical Nutrition* (2010), 91(6):1764–1768.

2.   Bazzano LA, He J, Ogden LG, et al. "Legume Consumption and Risk of Coronary Heart Disease in US Men and Women: NHANES I Epidemiologic Follow-Up Study." *Archives of Internal Medicine* (2001), 26; 161(21):2573–8.

3.   Vuksan V, Whitham D, Sievenpiper JL, et al. "Supplementation of Conventional Therapy with the Novel Grain Salba (*Salvia hispanica L.*) Improves Major and Emerging Cardiovascular Risk Factors in Type 2 Diabetes." *Diabetes Care* (2007), 30(11):2804–2810.

4.   Khan A, Safdar M, Ali Khan MM, et al. "Cinnamon Improves Glucose and Lipids of People with Type 2 Diabetes." *Diabetes Care* (2003), 26(12):3215–3218.

5.   *American Heart Association.* "Fish and Omega-3 Fatty Acids." Accessed May 7, 2010. http://www.americanheart.org/presenter.jhtml?identifier=4632

6.   *U.S. Environmental Protection Agency.* "What You Need to Know about Mercury in Fish and Shellfish." Accessed May 7, 2010. http://www.epa.gov/fishadvisories/advice/

7.   *U.S. Environmental Protection Agency.* Reports and Chemical Fact Sheets. Public Health Implications Of Exposure To Polychlorinated Biphenyls (PCBs). Accessed May 6, 2010. http://www.epa.gov/fishadvisories/technical/pcb99.html

8.   *Environmental Defense Fund.* "Health Alerts." Accessed May 12, 2010. http://www.edf.org/page.cfm?tagID=15904

9.   Kuriyama S, Shimazu T, Ohmori K, et al. "Green Tea Consumption and Mortality Due to Cardiovascular Disease, Cancer, and All Causes in Japan." *Journal of the American Medical Association* (2006), 296(10):1255–1265.

10. *U.S. Department of Health and Human Services. Food and Drug Administration.*
"Federal Register 62 FR 15343, March 31, 1997 — Food Labeling: Health Claims;
Soluble Fiber from Whole Oats and Risk of Coronary Heart Disease; Final Rule."
Accessed May 15, 2010. http://www.fda.gov/Food/LabelingNutrition/LabelClaims/
HealthClaimsMeetingSignificantScientificAgreementSSA/ucm074514.htm

11. Erkkila AT, Herrington DM, Mozaffarian D, et al. "Cereal Fiber and Whole-Grain
intake Are Associated with Reduced Progression of Coronary-Artery Atherosclerosis in
Postmenopausal Women with Coronary Artery Disease." *American Heart Journal* (2005),
150(1):94–101.

12. *U.S. Department of Health and Human Services. Food and Drug Administration.*
"Qualified Health Claims. April 2008." Accessed May 15, 2010. http://www.fda.gov/Food/
GuidanceComplianceRegulatoryInformation/GuidanceDocuments/FoodLabelingNutrition/
FoodLabelingGuide/ucm064923.htm

13. Covas, MI. "Olive Oil and the Cardiovascular System." *Pharmacological Research* (2007),
55(3):175–186.

14. *National Archives and Records Administration.* "Electronic Code of Federal Regulations,
101.83 Health Claims: Plant Sterol/Stanol Esters and Risk of Coronary Heart Disease
(CHD)." Accessed May 20, 2010. http://ecfr.gpoaccess.gov/cgi/t/text/text-idx?c=ecfr;sid=c41
5b1af63eade20b4a3991ce384d942;rgn=div8;view=text;node=21%3A2.0.1.1.2.5.1.14;idno=2
1;cc=ecfr

15. *U.S. Department of Health & Human Services. U.S. Food and Drug Administration.* "Federal
Register 64 FR 57699 October 26, 1999 — Food Labeling: Health Claims; Soy Protein and
Coronary Heart Disease; Final Rule." Accessed May 17, 2010. http://www.fda.gov/Food/
LabelingNutrition/LabelClaims/HealthClaimsMeetingSignificantScientificAgreementSSA/
ucm074740.htm

16. Zhan S and Ho SC. "Meta-Analysis of the Effects of Soy Protein Containing Isoflavones on
the Lipid Profile." *The American Journal of Clinical Nutrition* (2005), 81(2):397–408.

17. Messina MJ and Wood CE. "Soy Isoflavones, Estrogen Therapy, and Breast Cancer Risk:
Analysis and Commentary." *Nutrition Journal* (2008), 7:17.

18. Sesso HD, Liu S, Gaziano JM, et al. "Dietary Lycopene, Tomato-Based Food Products and
Cardiovascular Disease in Women." *The Journal of Nutrition* (2003), 133(6):2336–2341.

19. Sesso HD, Buring JE, Norkus EP, et al. "Plasma Lycopene, Other Carotenoids, and Retinol
and the Risk of Cardiovascular Disease in Women." *The American Journal Clinical Nutrition*
(2004), 79(1):47–53.

20. Lopez Ledesma R, Frati Munari AC, Hernandez Dominguez BC, et al. "Monounsaturated
Fatty Acid (Avocado) Rich Diet for Mild Hypercholesterolemia." *Archives of Medical
Research* (1996), 27(4): 519–523.

21. Mink PJ, Scrafford CG, Barraj LM, et al. "Flavonoid Intake and Cardiovascular Disease
Mortality: A Prospective Study in Postmenopausal Women." *The American Journal Clinical
Nutrition* (2007), 85(3):895–909.

22. Mostofsky E, Levitan EB, Wolk A, et al. "Chocolate Intake and Incidence of Heart Failure: A
Population-Based Prospective Study of Middle-Aged and Elderly Women." *Circulation Heart
Failure* (2010), 3:612-616.

23. Wu JN, Ho SC, Zhou C, et al. "Coffee consumption and risk of coronary heart diseases: A
Meta-Analysis of 21 Prospective Cohort Studies." *International Journal of Cardiology* (2009),
137(3):216–225.

24. Lopez-Garcia E, Rodriguez-Artalejo F, Rexrode KM, et al. "Coffee Consumption and Risk of Stroke in Women." *Circulation* (2009), 119(8):1067–1068.

25. Kelly JH and Sabaté J. "Nuts and Coronary Heart Disease: An Epidemiological Perspective." *British Journal of Nutrition* (2006), 96(Suppl 2):S61–S67.

26. *Office of Nutritional Products, Labeling and Dietary Supplements (2003-07-23).* "Qualified Health Claims: Letter of Enforcement Discretion — Nuts and Coronary Heart Disease (Docket No 02P-0505)." Center for Food Safety and Applied Nutrition. Archived from the original on 2008-06-17. http://web.archive.org/web/20080617172958/http://www.cfsan.fda.gov/~dms/qhcnuts2.html. Retrieved 2008-06-17

27. Lindberg, Matthew L.; Ezra A. Amsterdam. "Alcohol, Wine, and Cardiovascular Health." *Clinical Cardiology* (2008), 31(8): 347–351.

28. Khanna S, Roy S, Slivka A, et al. "Neuroprotective Properties of the Natural Vitamin E — Tocotrienol." *Stroke* (2005), 36(10):e144–e152.

Chapter 9

1. Gulati M, et al. "The Prognostic Value of a Nomogram for Exercise Capacity in Women." *The New England Journal of Medicine* (2005), 353(5):468–475.

2. Gulati M, et al. "Exercise Capacity and the Risk of Death in Women: The St James Women Take Heart Project." *Circulation* (2003), 108(13):1554–1559.

3. See #1

4. Mosca, L et al. "Evidence-Based Guidelines for Cardiovascular Disease Prevention in Women: 2007 Update." *Circulation* (2007), 115(11):1481–1501.

5. Haskell WL, et al. "Physical Activity and Public Health: Updated Recommendations from the American College of Sports Medicine and the American Heart Association." *Circulation* (2007), 116(9):1081–1093.

6. Nelson ME, et al. "Physical Activity and Public Health in Older Adults." *Circulation* (2007), 116(9):1094–1105

7. *Division of Nutrition, Physical Activity and Obesity, National Center for Chronic Disease Prevention and Health Promotion.* "2008 Physical Activity Guidelines for Americans." Accessed August 25, 2010. http://www.health.gov/paguidelines/guidelines/summary.aspx

8. *Canada's Physical Activity Guide, Public Health Agency of Canada.* Accessed October 4, 2010. http://www.phac-aspc.gc.ca/hp-ps/hl-mvs/pag-gap/index-home-accueil-eng.php

Chapter 10

1. *American Psychological Association.* "Mind-Body Health: Did You Know?" Accessed March 20, 2010. http://www.apa.org/helpcenter/mind-body.aspx

2. *American Psychological Association.* "Stress in America poll." Accessed October 24, 2007. www.apa.org/pubs/info/reports/2007-stress.doc

3. Levi, L. "Occupational Stress: Spice of Life or Kiss of Death?" *American Psychologist* (1990), 45(10):1142–1145.

4. *American Psychological Association.* "Stress in America poll." Accessed October 24, 2007. www.apa.org/pubs/info/reports/2007-stress.doc

5. Ibid.

6. *United States Department of Labor, Women's Bureau.* "Quick Stats on Women Workers, 2008." Accessed April 19, 2010. http://www.dol.gov/wb/stats/main.htm

7. Statistics Canada, "Women in Canada: Work Chapter Updates." Accessed November 26, 2010. http://www.statcan.gc.ca/pub/89f0133x/89f0133x2006000-eng.htm

8. Navaie-Waliser M, Feldman PH, Gould D A, et al. "When the Caregiver Needs Care: The Plight of Vulnerable Caregivers." *American Journal of Public Health* (2002), 92(3):409–13.

9. *National Center on Caregiving, Family Caregiver Alliance.* "Selected Caregiver Statistics." Accessed March 26, 2010. http://www.caregiver.org/caregiver/jsp/content_node. jsp?nodeid=439

10. Ibid.

11. Frasure-Smith N and Lesperance F. "Depression and Other Psychological Risks Following Myocardial Infarction." *Archives of General Psychiatry* (2003), 60(6):627–636.

12. Kubzansky LD, Davidson KW, Rozanski A. "The Clinical Impact of Negative Psychological States: Expanding the Spectrum of Risk for Coronary Artery Disease." *Psychosomatic Medicine* (2005), 67(Suppl 1):S10–S14.

13. Rosengren A, Hawken S, Ounpuu S, Sliwa K, Zubaid M, Almahmeed WA, Blackett KN, Sitthi-Amorn C, Sato H, Yusuf S. "Association of Psychosocial Risk Factors with Risk of Acute Myocardial Infarction in 11119 cases and 13648 Controls from 52 countries (The INTERHEART Study): Case–Control Study." *The Lancet* (2004), 364(9438):953–962.

14. Niaura R, Todaro JF, Stroud L, et al. "Hostility, the Metabolic Syndrome, and Incident Coronary Heart Disease." Health Psychology (2002), 21(6):588–593.

15. Tindle HA, Chang YF, Kuller LH, et al. "Optimism, Cynical Hostility, and Incident Coronary Heart Disease and Mortality in the Women's Health Initiative." *Circulation* (2009), 120(8):656–662.

16. Black, PH. "Stress and the Inflammatory Response: A Review of Neurogenic Inflammation." *Brain, Behavior, and Immunity* (2002), 16(6):622–653; Black, PH. "The Inflammatory Response Is an Integral Part of the Stress Response: Implications for Atherosclerosis, Insulin Resistance, Type II Diabetes and Metabolic Syndrome X." *Brain, Behavior, and Immunity* (2003), 17(5):350–364; and Black, PH and Garbutt, LD. "Stress, Inflammation and Cardiovascular Disease." *Journal of Psychosomatic Research* (2002), 52(1):1–23.

17. Toker S, Shirom A, Shapira I, et al. "The Association Between Burnout, Depression, Anxiety, and Inflammation Biomarkers: C-Reactive Protein and Fibrinogen in Men and Women." *Journal of Occupational Health Psychology* (2005), 10(4):344–362.

18. Hallman T, Burell G, Setterlind S, et al. "Psychosocial Risk Factors for Coronary Heart Disease, Their Importance Compared with Other Risk Factors and Gender Differences in Sensitivity." *Journal of Cardiovascular Risk* (2001), 8(1):39–49.

19. Slopen N, Glynn RJ, Buring J, Albert MA. "Job Strain, Job Insecurity, and Incident Cardiovascular Disease in the Women's Health Study." *Circulation* (2010), 122(20):A18520.

20. Wittstein IS, Thiemann DR, Lima JA, et al. "Neurohumoral Features of Myocardial Stunning Due to Sudden Emotional Stress." *The New England Journal of Medicine* (2005), 352(6):539–548.

21.   Auddy B, Hazra J, Mitra A, et al. "A Standardized Withania Somnifera Extract Significantly Reduces Stress-Related Parameters in Chronically Stressed Humans: A Double-Blind, Randomized, Placebo-Controlled Study." *The Journal of the American Nutraceutical Association* (2008), 11(1):50–56.

22.   Burt CW, Bernstein AW. "Observations from the CDC: Trends in Use of Medications Associated with Women's Ambulatory Care Visits." *Journal of Women's Health* (2003), 12(3):213–217.

23.   Guo X, Zhou B, Nishimura T, et al. "Clinical Effect of Qigong Practice on Essential Hypertension: A Meta-Analysis of Randomized Controlled trials." *Journal of Alternative and Complementary Medicine* (2008), 14(1):27–37.

Chapter 11

1.   *National Sleep Foundation.* "Sleep in America Poll, 2007." Accessed March 29, 2010. http://www.sleepfoundation.org/sites/default/files/Summary_Of_Findings%20-%20FINAL.pdf

2.   *National Sleep Foundation.* "Sleep in America Poll, 2009." Accessed March 29, 2010. http://www.sleepfoundation.org/sites/default/files/2009%20Sleep%20in%20America%20SOF%20EMBARGOED.pdf

3.   McSweeney JC, Cody M, O'Sullivan P, et al. "Women's Early Warning Symptoms of Acute Myocardial Infarction." *Circulation* (2003), 108(21):2619–2623.

4.   Ayas NY, White DP, Manson JE, et al. "A Prospective Study of Sleep Duration and Coronary Heart Disease in Women." *Archives of Internal Medicine* (2003), 163(2):205–209.

5.   Cappuccio FP, Stranges S, Kandala NP. "Gender-Specific Associations of Short Sleep Duration With Prevalent and Incident Hypertension: The Whitehall II Study." *Hypertension* (2007), 50(4):693–700.

6.   King CR, Knutson KL, Rathouz PJ, et al. "Short Sleep Duration and Incident Coronary Artery Calcification." *The Journal of the American Medical Association* (2008), 300(24):2859–2866.

7.   Miller MA, Kandala NB, Kivimaki M, et al. "Gender Differences in the Cross-Sectional Relationships Between Sleep Duration and Markers of Inflammation: Whitehall II Study." *Sleep* (2009), 32(7):857–864.

8.   Chen JC, Brunner RL, Ren H, et al. "Sleep Duration and Risk of Ischemic Stroke in Postmenopausal Women." *Stroke* (2008), 39(12):3185–3192.

Chapter 12

1.   Lloyd-Jones DM, et al. "Heart Disease and Stroke Statistics — 2010 Update: A report from the American Heart Association." *Circulation* (2010), 121(7):e46–e215.

2.   Mosca L et al. "Twelve-Year Follow-Up of American Women's Awareness of Cardiovascular Disease Risk and Barriers to Heart Health." *Cardiovasc Qual Outcomes* (2010), 3(2):120–127.

3.   Daly C, et al. "Gender Differences in the Management and Clinical Outcome of Stable Angina." *Circulation* (2006), 113(4):490–498.

4.   Vaccarino V, et al. "Sex and Racial Differences in the Management of Acute Myocardial Infarction, 1994 through 2002." *The New England Journal of Medicine* (2005), 353(7):671–682.

5. Jani SM, et al. "Sex Differences in the Application of Evidence-Based Therapies for the Treatment of Acute Myocardial Infarction." *Archives of Internal Medicine* (2006), 166(11):1164–1170.

6. Alexander KP, et al. "Sex Differences in Major Bleeding with Glycoprotein IIb/IIIa Inhibitors." *Circulation* (2006), 114(13):1380–1387.

7. Vaccarino V, et al. "Sex Differences in Hospital Mortality after Coronary Artery Bypass Surgery. Evidence for a Higher Mortality in Younger Women." *Circulation* (2002), 105(10):1176–1181.

8. Vaccarino V, et al. "Gender Differences in Recovery after Coronary Artery Bypass Surgery." *Journal of the American College of Cardiology* (2003), 41(2):307–314.

9. Humphries KH, et al. "Significant Improvement in Short-Term Mortality in Women Undergoing Coronary Artery Bypass Surgery (1991 to 2004)." *Journal of the American College of Cardiology* (2007), 49(14). 1552–1558.

10. Puskas JD, et al. "Off-Pump Techniques Disproportionately Benefit Women and Narrow the Gender Disparity in Outcomes after Coronary Artery Bypass Surgery." *Circulation* (2007), 116(11 Suppl):I192–I199.

11. Birnie DH, Sambell C, Johansen H, et al. "Use of Implantable Cardioverter Defibrillators in Canadian and US Survivors of Out-of-Hospital Cardiac Arrest." *Canadian Medical Association Journal* (2007), 177(1):41–46.

12. Chou AF, et al. "Gender Disparities in the Quality of Cardiovascular Disease Care in Private Managed Care Plans. *Women's Health Issues* (2007), 17(3):120–130.

Resources

Chapter 5
American Heart Association
www.heart.org

Health Canada, Drug Product Database
http://www.hc-sc.gc.ca/dhp-mps/prodpharma/databasdon/index-eng.php

MedicineNet
www.medicinenet.com

National Institutes of Health, MedlinePlus
http://www.nlm.nih.gov/medlineplus/

Chapter 6
For more information on the DASH diet:
http://www.nhlbi.nih.gov/hbp/prevent/h_eating/h_eating.htm

Chapter 7
Health Canada, Natural Products Directorate
http://www.hc-sc.gc.ca/dhp-mps/prodnatur/index-eng.php

Linus Pauling Institute's Micronutrient Information Center
http://lpi.oregonstate.edu/infocenter/

National Institutes of Health, National Center for Complementary and Alternative Medicine
http://nccam.nih.gov/

National Institutes of Health, Office of Dietary Supplements
http://ods.od.nih.gov/

PDR Health
www.pdrhealth.com

Chapter 8
American Heart Association (information available on various diets, nutrition for heart health, tips on eating out, and much more)
www.heart.org

Canada's Food Guide, Health Canada
http://www.hc-sc.gc.ca/fn-an/food-guide-aliment/index-eng.php

Food Pyramid, United States Department of Agriculture
http://www.mypyramid.gov/

Heart and Stroke Foundation
www.heartandstroke.com

Chapter 9

Be Active Your Way (National Institutes of Health)
http://www.health.gov/paguidelines/pdf/adultguide.pdf

Canada's Physical Activity Guide to Healthy Active Living
http://www.phac-aspc.gc.ca/hp-ps/hl-mvs/pag-gap/index-home-accueil-eng.php

Evidence-Based Guidelines for Cardiovascular Disease Prevention in Women
http://circ.ahajournals.org/cgi/content/full/115/11/1481

Exercise during Pregnancy Guidelines
http://www.acog.org/publications/patient_education/bp119.cfm

Exercise Guideline by the American College of Sports Medicine
http://www.acsm.org/AM/Template.cfm?Section=Home_Page&TEMPLATE=CM/HTMLDisplay.cfm&CONTENTID=7764

Exercise Guidelines by the USA Center for Disease Control (CDC)
http://www.cdc.gov/physicalactivity/everyone/guidelines/index.html

Chapter 10

The American Institute of Stress
www.stress.org

The American Psychological Association
www.apa.org

Canadian Institute of Stress
www.stresscanada.org

Canadian Mental Health Association
www.cmha.ca

Chapter 11

American Psychological Association
www.apa.org

American Sleep Apnea Association
www.sleepapnea.org

Canadian Mental Health Association
www.cmha.ca

National Sleep Foundation
www.sleepfoundation.org

Index